Si King & Dave Myers
THE HAIRY
DIETERS
GOOD EATING

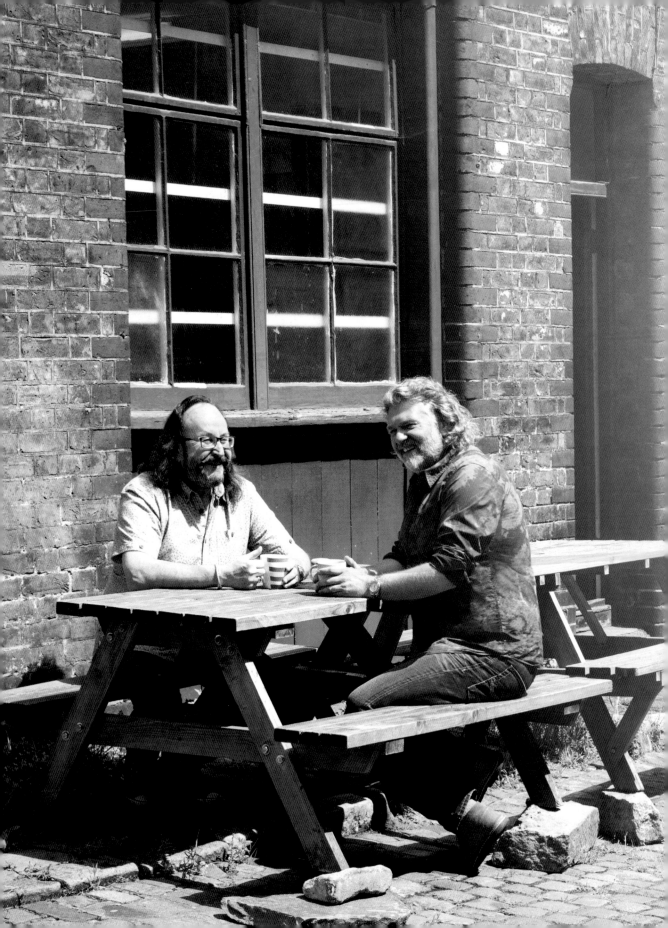

Si King & Dave Myers

THE HAIRY DIETERS

GOOD EATING

WEIDENFELD & NICOLSON

We'd like to dedicate this book to our families, to Ashley Adamson, Roy Taylor and their teams at Newcastle University who put us on the right path, and to all the lovely staff at the Royal Victoria Infirmary in Newcastle for helping us both so much when Si was poorly.

Si & Dave x

First published in Great Britain in 2014 by
Weidenfeld & Nicolson, an imprint of the Orion Publishing Group Ltd
Orion House, 5 Upper St Martin's Lane, London WC2H 9EA
An Hachette UK Company

10 9 8 7 6 5 4 3 2 1

A CIP catalogue record for this book is available from the British Library.

ISBN: 978 0 297 60898 1

Photographer: Andrew Hayes-Watkins
Food stylists: Anna Burges-Lumsden, Lisa Harrison
Food team: Phil Wells, Lucy O'Reilly, Jane Brown, Anna McManus
Editor: Jinny Johnson
Design and art direction: Loulou Clark
Technical artworker: Andy Bowden
Prop stylist: Loulou Clark
Proofreader: Elise See Tai
Indexer: Elizabeth Wiggans

Nutritional advice from Professor Ashley Adamson and Dr Suzana Almoosawi, Institute of Health & Society and Human Nutrition Research Centre, Newcastle University

Nutritional analysis calculated by:
Fiona Hunter, Bsc (Hons) Nutrition, Dip Dietetics

Printed and bound in Germany

The Orion Publishing Group's policy is to use papers that are natural, renewable and recyclable and made from wood grown in sustainable forests. The logging and manufacturing processes are expected to conform to the environmental regulations of the country of origin.

Every effort has been made to ensure that the information in this book is accurate. The information will be relevant to the majority of people but may not be applicable in each individual case, so it is advised that professional medical advice is obtained for specific health matters. Neither the publisher, authors or Optomen accept any legal responsibility for any personal injury or other damage or loss arising from the use or misuse of the information in this book. Anyone making a change in their diet should consult their GP, especially if pregnant, infirm, elderly or under 16.

optomen

CONTENTS

It's now more than two years since we started getting ourselves into shape and keeping our weight under control. We never thought it would happen, but the weight loss has really changed our attitude to cooking. We still enjoy eating as much as ever but we're more clued up, more aware of what we're putting in our mouths. And what's most important is that this hasn't taken the fun away at all – we're cooking great food that tastes fantastic and doesn't pile back the pounds. That's why we've called this latest collection of recipes Good Eating.

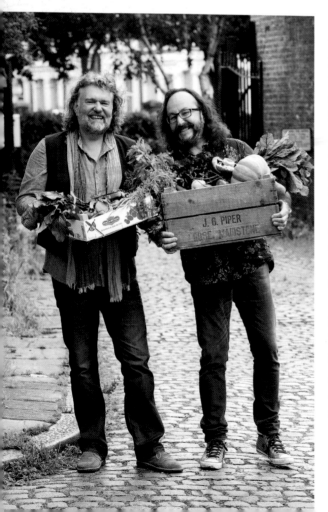

Back when we started dieting we had a lot of weight to lose and, as you know, we did it. And for the most part we've kept it off and we're both determined never to get that heavy again. We weigh ourselves regularly, and if the scales do show we've slipped a bit, we know it's a lot easier to shed two kilos than twenty.

It's made us realise that healthy eating really can be good eating and we wanted to know more. When we made our *Hairy Dieters* television series we worked with dietician and nutrition expert Professor Ashley Adamson at the University of Newcastle, who was a fantastic help to us. We decided to go back to her and chat through some questions that puzzled us and perhaps you too. Here's what we found out.

Si: **We hear a lot about low-carb diets and low-fat diets. Is it safe to cut down on carbs and fat at the same time?**
Ashley: What really matters is the quality of the carbohydrates and fats you eat. More complex carbs, such as those high in fibre, are good for you. Fats

such as monounsaturated and polyunsaturated fats are also good for you, but remember that **all** fat is high in calories. What you need to be thinking of is cutting out simple sugars (such as table sugar and fizzy drinks) as well as saturated or trans fats (lard, butter and the trans fats used in some ready-made cakes).

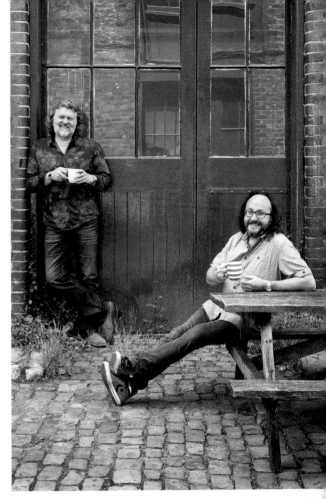

Foods high in simple sugars and saturated or trans fats are often low in nutrients but high in energy. They are what nutritionists often refer to as 'energy-dense' food. Energy-dense food is bad for you, compared to nutrient-dense foods (those containing vitamins and minerals), which are good for you. Examples of energy-dense foods are burgers, cakes, biscuits and confectionery. They give you few nutrients with a lot of energy (calories) in a small serving. Check the labels of some cakes and snacks and you will notice that although the portion might look small, the number of calories it contains can be surprising. Foods that are less processed or nearer to their natural form are less likely to be energy-dense. Nutrient-dense foods give you good value for your calories – that is, a lot of nutrients – and generally include foods such as vegetables and fruits and wholegrain cereals. For instance, a 100-gram bag of green leafy salad might only be 30 calories but provides you with lots of vitamins and minerals – it's good for you and you can eat a lot of it.

Dave: **People talk about good carbs and bad carbs but how do you know what's what? And what's the difference?**

Ashley: Good carbs are complex carbohydrates that contain plenty of fibre – food such as whole grains, vegetables and pulses. The body absorbs these slowly, meaning it takes time to break them down and release the sugars slowly into your system. Bad or simple carbs contain refined sugars – think biscuits, jams, soft drinks, sweets. These are bad because your body absorbs them quickly, which creates sugar surges in your blood. The more your blood sugar levels go up and down, the more harmful it is for your body. Our body doesn't like the yo-yo effect caused by these foods.

Si: Why is olive oil seen as better for you than lard, even though it contains as many calories? What are good fats and bad fats? And what are trans fats?

Ashley: Olive oil is high in monounsaturated and polyunsaturated fats. Lard and butter are high in saturated fat, while some margarines and spreads contain trans fat and others are high in polyunsaturated or monounsaturated fats. Both saturated and trans fats are known to be bad for your heart because they can make your blood thick and more likely to clot. Monounsaturated and polyunsaturated fats, on the other hand, make your blood more fluid, meaning you are less likely to develop blood clots.

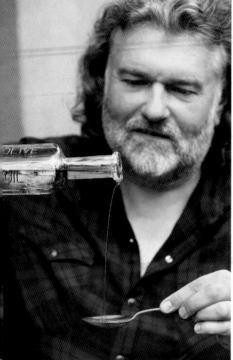

Our brain and nervous system are made mainly out of fat, which is why it is important to have some good fats, such as olive oil, in your diet. But it's important to remember that some oils are not designed for cooking. If you want to stir-fry your vegetables or roast them, opt for rapeseed oil or sunflower oil. Both these oils are high in monounsaturated fat and have a high burning point, which means they don't generate harmful substances if you overheat your pan. Olive oil is rich in polyunsaturated fats, which are good for your heart. However, it's best to reserve the use of extra virgin oil as a dressing for salads. It has a lower burning point than some other oils so might not be ideal for roasting or stir-frying.

Dave: We know we should be watching our sugar intake but how can we cut down? What should we look out for when shopping?

Ashley: When a food claims to be low-fat, beware – it may be high in sugar so check the ingredient list. Sucrose, maltose, dextrose, glucose, fructose, fruit sugar and ingredients such as honey, concentrated fruit juice and corn syrup are all just other names for added sugar. New guidelines recommend that no more than 5 per cent of our calories should come from added sugar. Given that most of us have about 14 per cent, that's a lot of sugar to cut out, but give it a go and you'll feel better for it.

Si: Are sugar substitutes safe? Which are the best ones?

Ashley: Artificial sweeteners and sweeteners such as aspartame, saccharin and stevia are all permitted and declared safe by the UK Food Standards Agency and the EU. They are lower in calories than sugar but using these sweeteners doesn't help you to kick the habit of eating sweet foods. It's far better to cut down on sweet stuff overall and have the occasional treat – you'll find the less you have the less you want. The more regulated your sugar level, the less likely you are to feel exhausted or down. Encourage children to drink water, milk or very dilute pure fruit juice instead of carbonated drinks, even if they are diet versions or sugar-free.

Dave: **What about the sugar in fruit and fruit juices? Is that OK?**

Ashley: Fruit and fruit juice contain vitamins and minerals as well as naturally occurring sugars so they're not as bad as sugary drinks like orange squash, cola and lemonade. Those are basically sugar and water with a few flavourings. But remember that pure fruit juice contains a similar amount of sugar to non-diet drinks, such as colas, so if you're drinking juice regularly you can end up taking in too many calories in the form of sugar. It's better to eat whole fruit as it is and drink plain water or other beverages such as tea, herbal or fruit teas, or milk (ideally, 1 per cent-fat milk) to keep your body hydrated.

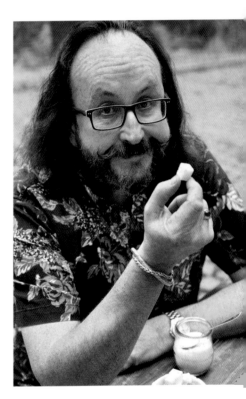

In general, we find it easier to take calories as liquids rather than solids. Our stomach also digests liquids quicker, meaning that you might end up drinking more (so taking in more calories) and being hungry quicker when consuming liquids compared to solid food.

Si: **Is brown bread better for us than white sliced and why?**

Ashley: This is an interesting question, as people often confuse wholemeal bread with brown bread, some of which is simply white flour dyed with caramel to add colour. It's wholemeal bread – bread with bits in – that we should generally eat, as it is high in fibre and contains a variety of vitamins and minerals. If you really don't like wholemeal bread, the next best are the newer half and half breads. As before when we talked about avoiding energy-dense foods, there's a concept in nutrition called 'nutrient density'. In general, foods that provide more nutrients for the same amount of calories are described as nutrient-dense and considered healthiest, as they help us avoid consuming empty calories. So the next time you eat something ask yourself: what does this food give me other than calories? As a rough guide, if it provides lots of important minerals or vitamins you know that it is probably good for you.

Dave: **I love salt. I know it's bad for my heart and blood pressure but will eating salty foods affect my weight?**

Ashley: Many salty foods, such as crisps and peanuts, are also high in fat so contain lots of calories – they're energy-dense – so it's best to limit your intake. In cooking, try using less salt or none at all and use lovely herbs and spices for flavour instead – I know you do this in lots of your recipes. Try covering up some of the holes on your salt shaker so you don't put so much on your food. You will be surprised that your taste buds will get used to less salt – really.

Si: **How much water should I drink every day?**

Ashley: The European Food Safety Authority advises that women should drink about 1.6 litres of fluid and men about 2.0 litres of fluid per day. That's equivalent to eight 200ml glasses for a woman and ten 200ml glasses for a man. This could be in the form of tea, herbal/fruit teas, coffee, milk (semi-skimmed or 1 per cent-fat milk) or the occasional fruit juice.

Dave: **What about exercise for weight loss? How many tangos do I need to do to work off a bag of crisps or a chocolate bar?**

Ashley: The current recommendation for adults is 30 minutes of moderate physical activity at least five times a week. When you think of it in terms of food, one standard Mars bar = 50 minutes of aqua aerobics, while just three minutes of dancing burns off the calories in a carrot, and 16 minutes of walking = one banana.

Some people have intense gym workouts on a couple of days, then think it's fine to spend the rest of the time lying on the sofa watching television. This is what some scientists refer to as being an 'active couch potato'. It's best to distribute exercise through the day and be less sedentary if you want to reduce your risk of developing diabetes or high blood pressure. If you're working in an office, take a short break every hour to stretch or walk down to the water cooler. Walking is good exercise and free. Why drive to the gym when you can walk to work or the shops?

Si: **Can we eat our five a day and still lose weight?**

Ashley: If you snack on fruit and veg and include plenty in your main meals, you'll have less room for unhealthy snacks such as crisps, cakes and pies in your diet, so that's good for weight control.

Fruit and vegetables are generally lower in calories than foods such as dairy products, meats and cereals. When selecting your fruit and vegetables, choose some with a high water content, such as berries, watermelons, pineapples, cucumbers, green leafy vegetables, and tomatoes. These are generally rich in vitamins but low in calories – that is, they have a low energy density but high nutrient density. This means you are more likely to get all the vitamins and minerals you need in fewer calories so encouraging weight loss.

Dave: **Will I lose more weight if I eat more fibre and go to the loo more often?**

Ashley: Some types of fibre help your body get rid of some fat (cholesterol) and gets it out of your system. More importantly, fibre helps you feel full for longer and keeps those hunger pangs at bay. Foods high in fibre tend to be complex carbohydrates and so take longer for your body to digest and avoid that yo-you effect. It doesn't necessarily mean you'll be spending all your time in the toilet, though. It just helps improve your digestive system so you don't get constipated (no fun for anyone) and have more regular bowel movements.

Si: **Sometimes I don't feel like eating breakfast but should I have some anyway? Is it true that you need to eat something in the morning to get your metabolism going?**

Ashley: People with high levels of stress hormones and insulin resistance tend to have a lower appetite in the morning and want to eat more later in the day. Because eating later in the day is related to weight gain, continuing this pattern of eating will create a continuous cycle wherein you increase your body's stress hormones, which makes you want to skip breakfast and eat later in the day. This in turn increases your stress hormones and so on. Think of your body as a clock. From time to time, our body clock goes off track and we need to reset it in order to allow our metabolism to function better. If you encourage yourself to have breakfast every day, even if it's just a light snack or a piece of fresh fruit, then over time you will notice that your metabolism will reset itself and you'll start craving more food in the morning and less in the evening.

Dave: **I've heard people talk about visceral fat. What is this and can thin people have it?**

Ashley: Visceral fat is belly fat – the fat we put on round our waists and our organs (inside fat). There's good evidence that the larger our waistlines the higher our risk of conditions such as heart disease and cancers. This is why keeping a check on our waist measurement as well as our body weight is important. As a general rule, in men a waist measurement of more than 102cm is considered to be unhealthy, while in women a waist measurement above 88cm is likely to be linked with health problems. The different cut-offs are related to the fact that men are more likely to have an apple shape and gain weight easily around the abdomen, while women are more likely to have a pear shape, and gain weight around the hips. Just another of our many differences! If your waist measurement is above these numbers your health could be at risk. Your waist measurement is easy to keep track of too – we all know when we've had to move to the next notch on our belts or those trousers seem to have 'shrunk in the wash'!

Si: **When you look at a food packet there are usually two measurements for calories. One is more than the other, so which should we be looking at?**

Ashley: Both measure the amount of energy we are putting in our bodies but they are different units (like inches and centimetres). Kj (kilojoules) are equal to just over four times kcal (kilocalories – sometimes called just calories). Checking your kcal is easier because we often hear nutritional recommendations in calories.

It's difficult to give precise calorie recommendations because we are all different sizes and have varying levels of activity. Think of types of cars – some are minis, others are big four-wheel drives. Neither uses much petrol just to idle at the roadside but they need different amounts of petrol to drive 50 miles. In the UK, on average, men are recommended to have a maximum of about 2,500 kcal and women 2,000 kcal, though this varies depending on body size and activity levels (how many calories you burn). Remember, though, this is a guide, not a goal.

Keep in mind that some food labels show only a rough estimate of the calories they contain, so the bowl of cereal or muffin you're eating might have a few more calories than you think. Also remember to check the serving size. You might think the calorie count is for a whole packet but it could be for only a portion of it. If you want to lose weight, then you need to eat less than your body uses (burns). As a rough guide, if your weight is currently stable and you eat about 500 calories less each day for a week you'll lose about 500 grams a week or a kilo in two weeks.

QUICK TIPS

We've given calorie counts (in kilocalories) for all our recipes so follow the recipes carefully so you don't change the calorie count. Weigh your ingredients and use proper spoons and a measuring jug. We always say how many people the recipe will serve, so u don't eat more than your fair share!

We mention spray oil in quite a few of the recipes, as this is an easy way of reducing the amount of oil you use. Buy the most natural kind you can find and spritz it lightly. If you don't want to use spray oil, just brush on a small amount of oil.

Peel onions and garlic unless otherwise specified. Use fresh stock or stock made with a cube, as you prefer. And we use free-range eggs and chicken whenever possible. We've also highlighted recipes suitable for freezing. Follow the usual safety advice when defrosting and reheating.

BREAKFAST AND BRUNCH

We're much more adventurous with our breakfasts now than we used to be. We still love our eggs, but instead of a fry-up we might go for a delicious frittata-style omelette stuffed with fresh veg, or some little pots of baked eggs with different fillings. When time is short, we both love a smoothie, which gives you loads of goodness in a matter of minutes and really keeps you going. And for a special treat, try our fab ham, corn and chilli muffins. They're awesome!

AMERICAN-STYLE FLUFFY PANCAKES

135 calories per portion (3 pancakes)

These little morning lovelies are usually made with ricotta but we use quark. This is nought to do with ducks but is a low-fat dairy product available in most supermarkets, which takes the calorie count of the pancakes right down. Enjoy them with some low-fat yoghurt or crème fraiche and some extra berries. You can also drizzle on a little maple syrup – a teaspoonful only adds about 15 calories. We're sure you won't need any encouragement, but eat these as soon as they're cooked to enjoy them at their very best.

Serves 4 (3 pancakes each)
Prep: 10 minutes
Cooking time: 12 minutes

100g plain flour
1 tsp baking powder
50g quark
125g semi-skimmed milk
2 egg whites
100g blueberries
oil, for spraying

Sift the flour and baking powder into a large bowl. In a separate bowl, mix the quark and milk until fairly smooth. Add a little of the quark mixture to the flour to make a fairly thick paste, then use an electric mixer to gradually incorporate the rest.

In a clean bowl, whisk the egg whites until they form dry, stiff peaks. Using a metal spoon, fold 2 tablespoons of the egg whites into the batter to loosen it a little. Gently fold in the rest, being careful not to knock the air out of the mixture. Stir the blueberries into the batter.

Heat a large non-stick frying pan over a medium heat, then give it one quick spray of oil. Dollop large spoonfuls of the batter into the frying pan – you should be able to cook at least 3 at once. When you see lots of little air bubbles breaking through on the surface of the pancakes and the batter is starting to look as though it is setting, flip each one over and cook for another minute. Remove and set aside to keep warm.

Continue to cook the rest of the pancakes in the same way, then serve immediately.

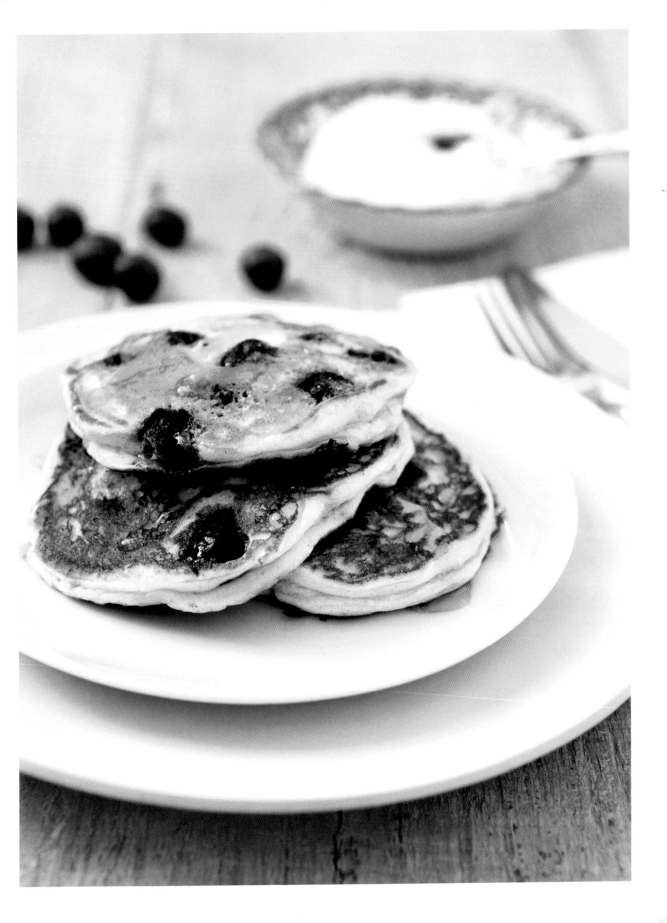

BUCKWHEAT PANCAKES

75 calories per pancake; 193 calories with filling

Buckwheat flour makes great pancakes – known as galettes to our friends in Brittany – and it's available in most supermarkets. Despite the name, it's not actually a wheat and it's gluten free so is good for those with wheat allergies. The batter uses one egg and makes eight pancakes – more than you need – but it freezes well or can be kept in the fridge for a few days.

Serves 4
Prep: 15 minutes, plus an hour standing time for the batter if possible
Cooking time: 15 minutes

Pancakes
100g buckwheat flour
1 pinch of salt
1 large egg
300ml semi-skimmed milk
oil, for spraying

Filling
1 tbsp olive oil
100g mushrooms, wiped clean and thinly sliced
1 garlic clove, finely chopped
1 tbsp finely chopped fresh parsley
4 eggs
flaked sea salt
freshly ground black pepper

FREEZE!

Pour any batter you don't use into an airtight plastic container and freeze for another time.

Sift the flour into a bowl and stir in the salt. Make a well in the flour and break in the egg, then gradually incorporate the flour into the egg until you have a thick paste. Start mixing in the milk, little by little, until you have a smooth batter. If you have time, leave the batter to stand for about an hour, but don't worry if you can't.

To make the filling, heat the oil in a non-stick frying pan and add the mushrooms. Fry until they are tender, then add the garlic and parsley. Season and cook for another minute or two, then tip everything into a bowl. Set the pan aside for cooking the eggs later.

To make the pancakes, heat a small non-stick frying pan over a medium heat and spritz lightly with oil. Hold the pan in one hand and add a small ladleful of batter (about 2 tablespoons), swirling quickly so the entire base of the pan is coated. Cook the pancake on one side until lots of little air bubbles appear and a palette knife slides easily under it. Flip the pancake over and cook on the other side for about half a minute, then slide on to a plate. Make 3 more pancakes in the same way. You shouldn't need to add more oil to the pan – the remaining pancakes will brown more quickly, but just turn down the heat a little and keep a close eye on them.

Break the eggs into the pan you used to cook the mushrooms and fry gently until the whites are set and the yolks are still runny.

Return a pancake to the pancake pan. Put a quarter of the mushrooms in the centre and top with a fried egg. Turn the edges of the pancake into the centre – they won't meet so you'll see the filling peeking through the gap. Transfer to a warm plate. Fill the rest of the pancakes in the same way and serve immediately.

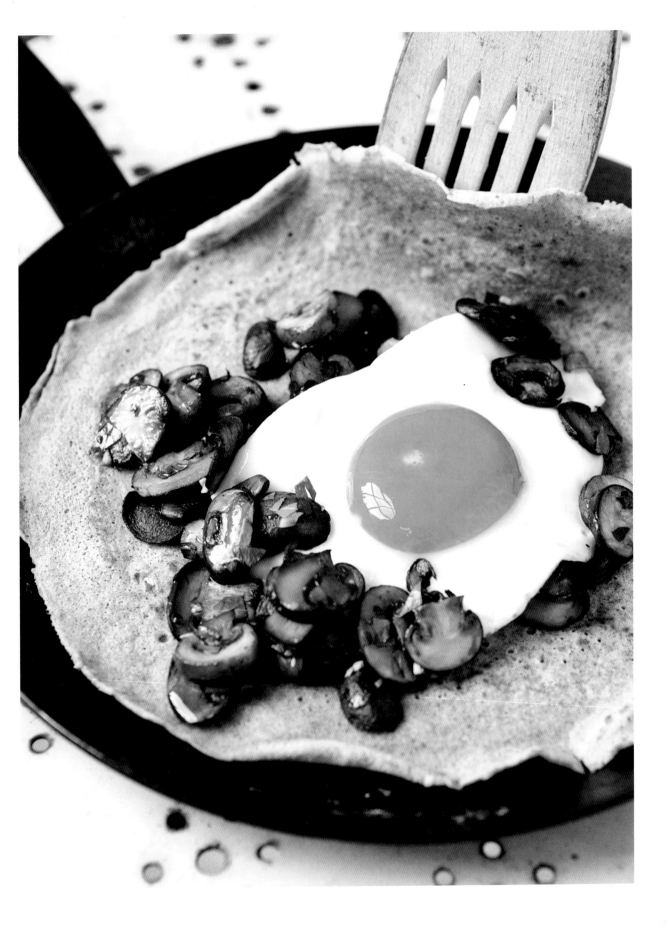

VEGETABLE FRITTATA

230 calories per portion

A frittata is basically a good hearty omelette that's finished off under the grill. We like to roast most of the veg for extra flavour and you can cook them the night before if you want a quick brunch dish for the morning. This dish is excellent cold too, so good for a lunch box or picnic basket. Vary the veg according to your taste and the season – asparagus, peas, mushrooms are all good – but stay way from the spuds and keep your calorie count in mind.

Serves 4
Prep: 15 minutes
Cooking time: 40 minutes

2 red onions, cut into wedges
1 courgette, cut into rounds
1 red pepper, deseeded and sliced
    lengthways into strips
200g butternut squash,
    peeled and diced
1 tbsp olive oil
1 tsp dried oregano
½ head of broccoli, broken into
    small florets
50g green beans, cut in half
6 eggs
oil, for spraying
6 cherry tomatoes, halved
handful of fresh basil leaves,
    torn
flaked sea salt
freshly ground black pepper

First roast the veg. Preheat the oven to 200°C/Fan 180°C/Gas 6. Line a baking tray or roasting dish with non-stick baking paper and spread the onions, courgette, red pepper and butternut squash over it. Drizzle on the olive oil, then turn the vegetables over with your hands, making sure they are all lightly coated with oil. Sprinkle with the oregano. Place the baking tray in the oven and roast the vegetables for 30 minutes, then set aside.

Bring a small saucepan of water to the boil and blanch the broccoli and beans for 2 minutes, then drain. Crack the eggs into a bowl, beat them with a fork and season with salt and pepper.

Heat your grill to its highest setting. Lightly spray a large non-stick frying pan with oil and place the pan over a medium heat. Tip the roasted veg into the frying pan and spread them out as evenly as you can so that each quarter gets a good balance of the different vegetables. Add the broccoli, green beans and cherry tomatoes and sprinkle over the torn basil.

Pour the eggs over the vegetables. Cook over a medium heat until the base of the frittata has set – you'll see the edges starting to turn brown. Place the frying pan under the hot grill and cook for a few more minutes until the eggs have set and the top of the frittata has started to puff up slightly. Remove carefully – the handle of the pan will be hot – cut into quarters and serve.

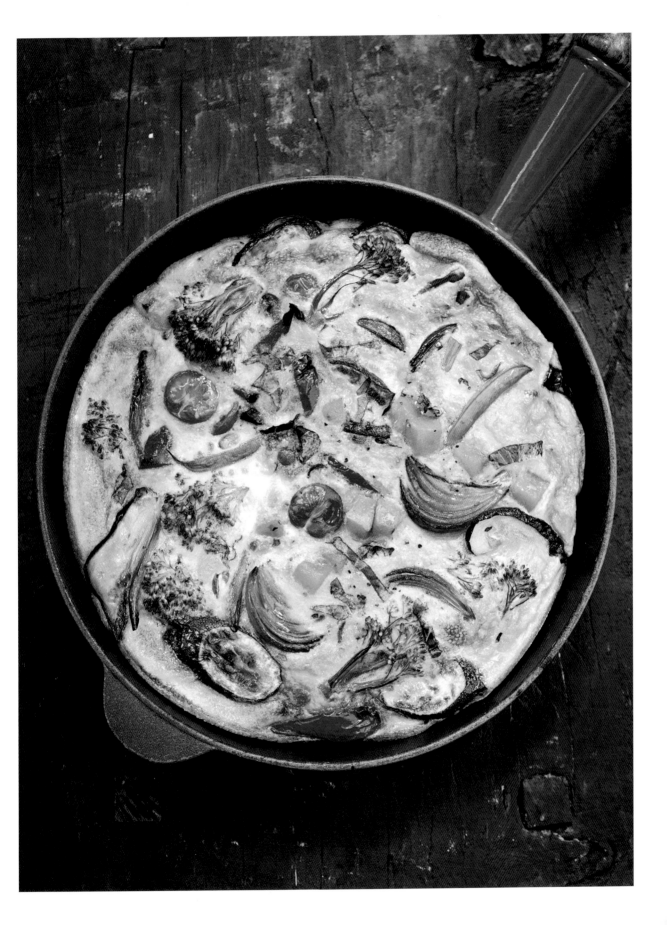

BAKED EGGS

155 calories per portion (with mushroom filling); 187 calories (with chorizo)

These make a really special breakfast or brunch with one of our fab fillings. We love chorizo and although it's high in calories, lots of the calorific oil comes out when you fry it. It's mega tasty too, so you don't need a lot.

Serves 4
Prep: 10 minutes
Cooking time: 15–20 minutes

oil, for spraying
4 large eggs
4 tsp finely grated Cheddar,
    Gruyère or other hard cheese
flaked sea salt
freshly ground black pepper

Mushroom filling
1 tbsp olive oil
4 button mushrooms, wiped and
    finely sliced
1 garlic clove, finely chopped
4 squares of frozen spinach,
    defrosted and liquid squeezed out
a grating of nutmeg

Chorizo filling
50g chorizo, finely chopped
½ red pepper, deseeded and
    finely chopped
½ onion, finely chopped
1 garlic clove, finely chopped
4 tomatoes, roughly chopped
basil leaves, shredded

Preheat the oven to 190°C/Fan 170°C/Gas 5. Very lightly mist 4 ramekins with oil. Choose your filling and prepare as below, then divide the filling between the ramekins. Break an egg into each ramekin, on top of the filling, and season with salt and pepper. Sprinkle a teaspoon of cheese over each egg and cover each ramekin with foil.

Put the ramekins in a roasting or baking dish and pour in hot water to come about two-thirds up the sides of the ramekins. Bake in the oven for up to 15 minutes, checking them after 10 minutes. You can cook the eggs to your liking, but after about 10 minutes the whites should be set and the yolks should still be runny.

Mushroom filling
Heat the olive oil in a frying pan, add the mushrooms and cook them until soft. Add the garlic and season with salt and pepper, then cook for another minute. Make sure the spinach is as dry as possible before adding it to the mushrooms in the pan. Grate over a little nutmeg and stir well to combine.

Chorizo filling
Put the chorizo in a frying pan and fry until brown – you don't need to add any extra oil, as the chorizo will immediately start giving out its own. Remove the chorizo and place it on some kitchen paper to drain, making sure there's only a very small amount of oil left in the frying pan. Add the red pepper and onion, then sauté until soft. Add the garlic and fry for another minute, then add the tomatoes. Cook for a few minutes until the tomatoes have reduced down slightly, then tip the chorizo back into the pan and stir in the basil.

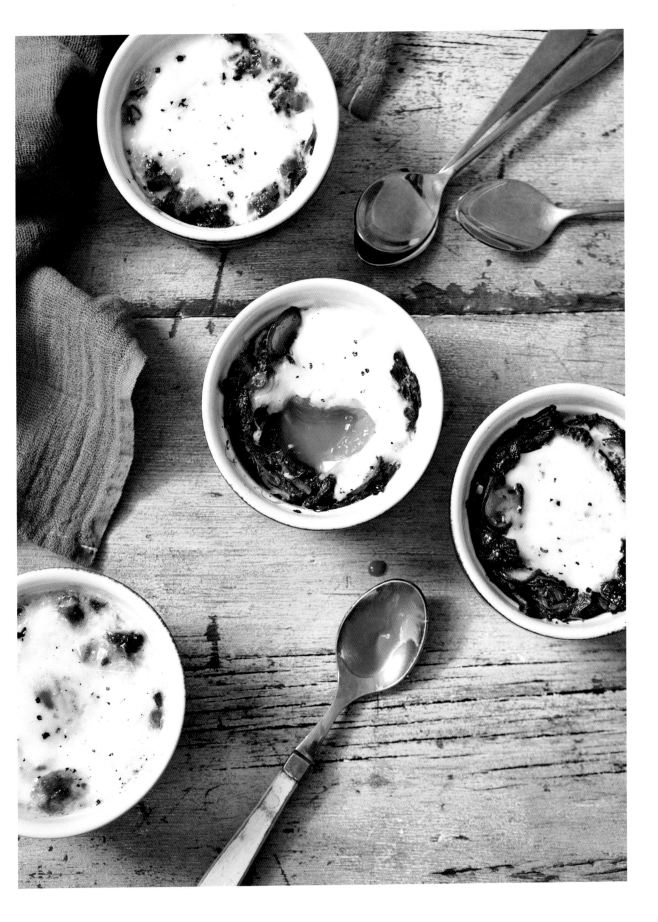

SMOOTHIES

70–104 calories per serving

Smoothies make a perfect breakfast treat or a quick pick-me-up at any time of day. We know we need fibre in our diet but sometimes it's nice to have a bit of smooth with the rough! It's so easy to make your own smoothies – some of the ready-made versions are expensive and can be full of calories.

Serves 2
Prep: 5–10 minutes

Green smoothie
50g spinach
1 celery stick
1 apple
juice of 1 orange
juice of 1 lime
½ tsp grated fresh root ginger
handful of ice cubes

Banana, strawberry and
blueberry smoothie
1 banana
100g strawberries
100g blueberries
50ml low-fat natural yoghurt
handful of ice cubes

Kiwi, nectarine and grape
smoothie
2 kiwi fruit
1 nectarine (or peach)
150g grapes
handful of ice cubes

Green smoothie (70 calories per serving)
Wash the spinach, roughly chop the celery and core and chop the apple. Put them into a blender with the rest of the ingredients. Blitz until smooth, then serve and drink right away.

Banana, strawberry and blueberry smoothie (103 calories per serving)
Peel the banana and hull the strawberries, then put them into a blender with the rest of the ingredients. Blitz until smooth, then serve and drink right away.

Kiwi, nectarine and grape smoothie (104 calories per serving)
Peel the kiwi fruit and remove the stone from the nectarine (or peach), then put them into a blender with the rest of the ingredients. Blitz until smooth, then serve and drink right away.

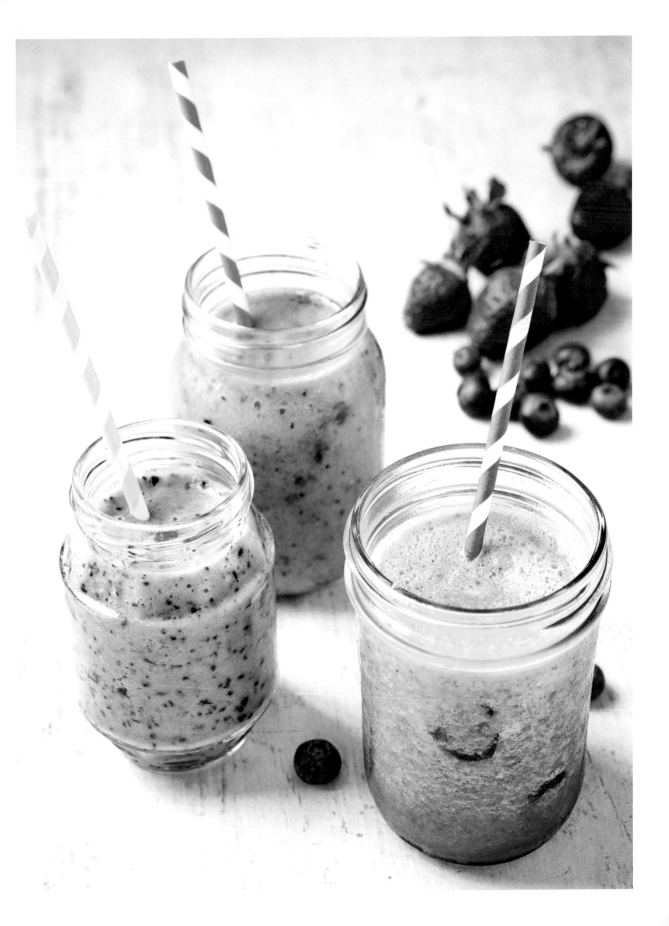

HAM, CORN AND CHILLI MUFFINS

120 calories per muffin

We've always loved the Texas cornbread we featured in Mums Know Best *and these muffins were inspired by that recipe. They make an awesome treat for brunch – or any time of day. We've cut right back on the fat in these and they still work really well, but do watch out for them sticking to the muffin cases. Best thing to do is to mist each case with a spray of oil.*

Makes 12
Prep: 15 minutes
Cooking time: 20 minutes

oil, for spraying
1 tsp lemon juice
250ml semi-skimmed milk
250g self-raising flour
2 tsp baking powder
1 tsp smoked paprika
½ tsp chilli powder
½ tsp dried oregano
50g Parma ham (or other well-
    flavoured ham), finely chopped
100g canned sweetcorn
2 medium eggs, beaten
25g reduced-fat Cheddar cheese,
    finely grated

Preheat the oven to 200°C/Fan 180°C/Gas 6. Line a muffin tin with paper cases and lightly spray each case with oil.

Add the lemon juice to the milk and leave it to stand for 5 minutes. It will thicken slightly and become similar to buttermilk.

Sift the flour, baking powder, smoked paprika and chilli powder into a large bowl. Add the dried oregano, chopped ham and sweetcorn, then mix everything together well.

Add the beaten eggs to the buttermilk and stir. Make a well in the centre of the flour mixture and pour in the wet ingredients. Stir just enough to combine, keeping the mixing to a minimum.

Spoon a heaped tablespoon of the mixture into each muffin case, then sprinkle some grated cheese over the top. Bake in the oven for 15–20 minutes until cooked. Remove the muffins from the oven and leave to cool – if you can resist them for that long!

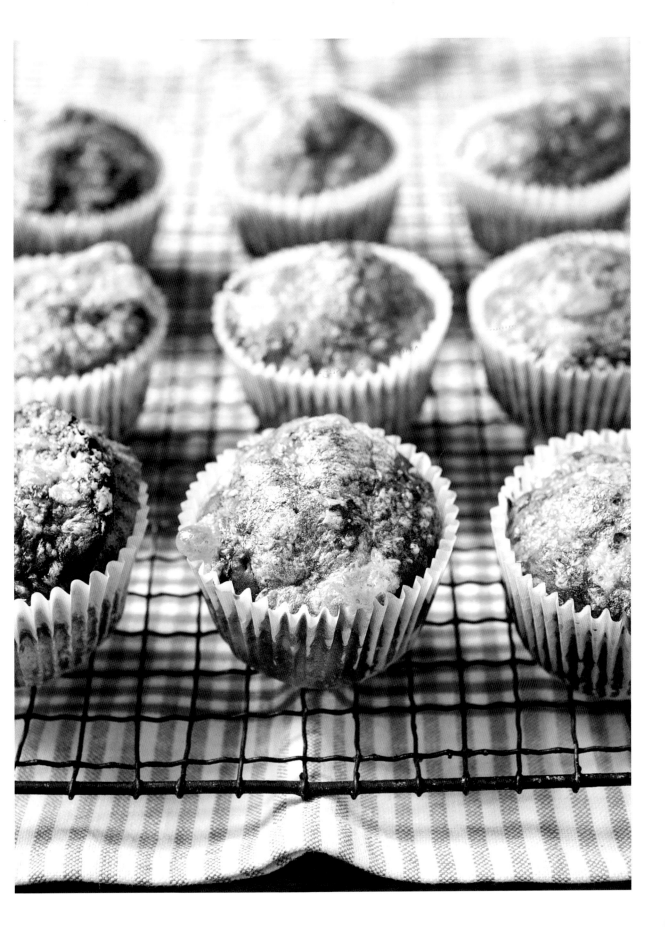

SMOKED HADDOCK OMELETTE

428 calories per portion (if serving 2); 285 calories per portion (if serving 3)

The idea for this recipe came from a dish known as omelette Arnold Bennett, after the famous novelist. It was created for him by the Savoy Hotel in London and became a much-loved classic. Our version is much less calorific than the original but is still very good to eat and surprisingly rich.

Serves 2–3
Prep: 20 minutes
Cooking time: 25 minutes

200g smoked haddock fillet
  (preferably undyed)
250ml semi-skimmed milk
1 tbsp cornflour
1 tbsp low-fat crème fraiche
1 tbsp finely chopped chives
oil, for spraying
5 eggs, beaten
25g reduced-fat Cheddar cheese,
  grated
freshly ground black pepper

Put the haddock in a wide saucepan and pour in the milk to cover. Bring to the boil, cover, then turn off the heat and leave to stand for 10 minutes. Strain the milk into a jug, then when the fish is cool enough to handle, break it up into chunks and set it aside. Discard the skin and any stray bones.

Mix the cornflour with a little cold water until you have a smooth paste. Measure 150ml of the cooking milk into a small saucepan and add the crème fraiche. Pour in the cornflour mixture and stir over a gentle heat until you have a thick sauce. Season with pepper, then stir in the haddock and the chives.

Heat a large frying pan and lightly spray it with oil. Pour in the beaten eggs, making sure the whole of the base of the frying pan is evenly covered. When the egg mixture is almost set, pile the haddock mixture over one half of the omelette and sprinkle the cheese on top. Carefully flip the uncovered half of the omelette over the filling and leave to cook for a couple of minutes until the cheese has melted.

Cut the omelette in half or divide into thirds and serve immediately.

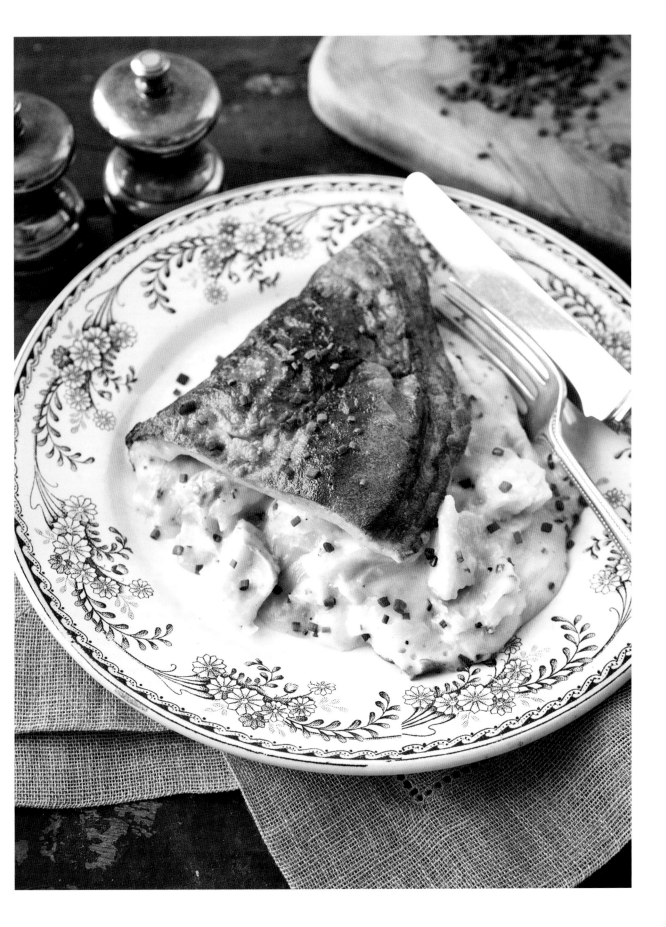

FAMILY FAVOURITES

Great family meals are at the heart of our cooking –
recipes that are good for those of us who need to shed
a pound or two but also keep the whole family happy.
We know that many people serve up the recipes from
our Hairy Dieters' books and the rest of the family enjoy
them so much they don't even realise that they are low
in calories! Honestly, since we've been writing the diet
books, these healthy dishes are what we cook for our
own families at home. In this chapter are some more
of our favourites for you to try, such as home-made fish
fingers, turkey chilli and some lip-smacking variations
on meatballs. Give 'em a go.

HOME-MADE BAKED BEANS

veggie: 103 calories per portion; bacon: 131 calories per portion

Everyone loves baked beans and our home-made version is extra tasty while cutting down on the sugar. This is best made with dried beans that you've soaked overnight, but you can whip it up with a couple of cans if need be. We like haricot beans, but you can use anything that takes your fancy. Check the packet for cooking times, though, if you do use different beans.

Serves 8 as a side dish
Prep: 15 minutes, plus soaking time
Cooking time: 1 hour 45 minutes

200g dried haricot or other
   beans (or 2 x 400g cans
   of cooked beans)
2 bay leaves
1 slice of onion
2 cloves
1 onion, very finely diced
1 carrot, peeled and very
   finely diced
1 celery stick, trimmed and very
   finely diced
1 tbsp vegetable oil
150ml vegetable stock
400g can of tomatoes
1 tbsp soy sauce
½ tsp sweet smoked paprika
pinch of ground cloves
flaked sea salt
freshly ground black pepper

Smoky bacon beans
½–1 tsp black treacle
100g smoked back bacon, fat
   trimmed and meat finely diced

If you're using dried beans, soak them overnight in plenty of cold water. Drain the beans, then put them in a large saucepan, add water to cover generously and bring to the boil. Keep skimming off any foam that forms until it turns white. Add the bay leaves, onion slice and cloves and continue to boil for 10 minutes, then turn the heat down and simmer for 45–60 minutes. The beans should be cooked through but not too soft, so check them regularly after 45 minutes. Drain, discarding the cooking liquid, bay, onion and cloves.

Meanwhile, prepare the vegetables. They should be chopped as finely as possible – almost to a purée – so you could use a food processor. Heat the oil in a saucepan, add the vegetables and cook them slowly for 10 minutes. Towards the end of this time, turn up the heat slightly so the vegetables start to caramelise – this adds sweetness to the sauce. Pour in the stock and simmer for 5 minutes, then add the tomatoes, soy sauce, paprika and cloves. Season and leave to simmer for about half an hour until the sauce is well reduced.

Using a stick blender or ordinary blender, purée the sauce until smooth. Tip it back into the pan, then add the beans (freshly cooked or canned). Simmer for 15 minutes to allow the flavours to blend.

Smoky bacon beans
Prepare the beans and veg as above, adding the treacle at the same time as the tomatoes and soy sauce. Start with half a teaspoon, simmer the sauce for a few minutes, then taste and add more treacle if you think it needs it. Fry the bacon in a non-stick frying pan until crisp and brown, then add it to the puréed sauce. Drain off any fat from the pan, then deglaze the pan with a little water and add this to the sauce too. Add the beans and simmer for 15 minutes as above.

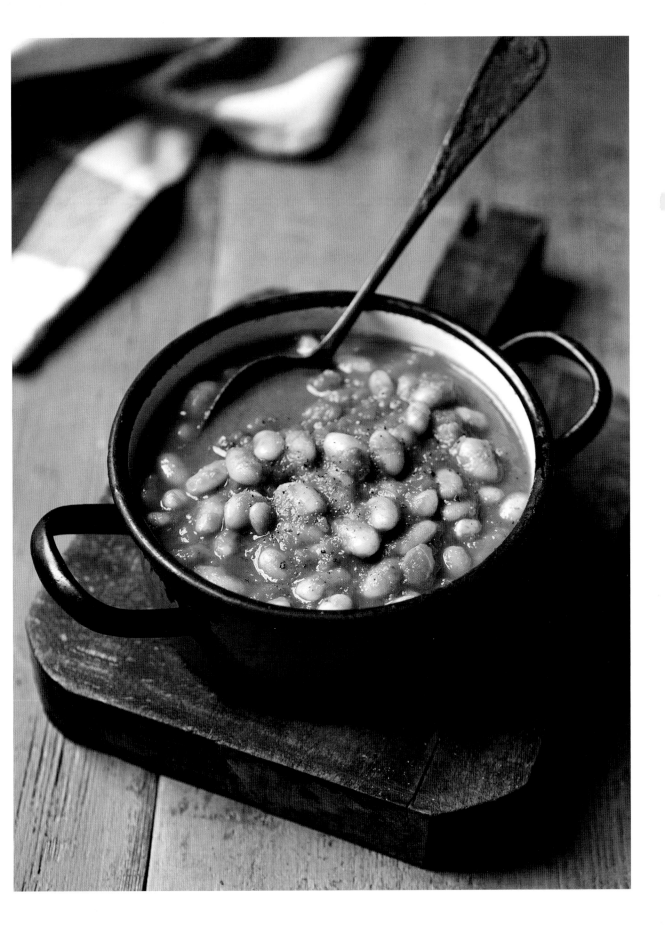

BUBBLE AND SQUEAK

107 calories per portion; 195 calories per portion with poached egg

There's nothing like a good bubble. In our recipe we've upped the carrot and swede and cut down on the potato so it's a bit lighter than usual but still tastes mega. Swede can go a bit mushy when boiled so we like to steam the veg, but if you don't have a steamer, just be sure to drain it all well. You could dry-fry the eggs if you prefer.

Serves 4
Prep: 15 minutes
Cooking time: 15–20 minutes

200g swede, peeled and diced
200g carrots, peeled and diced
200g potatoes, peeled and diced
200g cabbage, shredded
1 tsp olive oil
1 rasher of bacon, fat trimmed
  and meat finely diced
½ onion, finely chopped
4 eggs (optional)
1 tsp white wine vinegar (optional)
flaked sea salt
freshly ground black pepper

Layer the root vegetables in a steamer – swede on the bottom, carrots next, potatoes on top. Steam them over boiling water for 10 minutes or until all the vegetables are tender. If you don't have a steamer, boil the vegetables until tender, then drain them really well. Season the veg and then mash. You don't want the mixture to be too smooth, so don't be too vigorous about it.

Put the cabbage in a saucepan with a couple of centimetres of just-boiled water and simmer it for a few minutes until tender. Drain thoroughly. Add the olive oil to a large non-stick frying pan and fry the diced bacon until brown. Add the onion and cook until it is translucent and taking on a little colour. Tip the bacon and onion into the mash, along with the cabbage, and stir.

Heat the grill to its highest setting. Pile all the mixture into the frying pan and cook over a medium heat for several minutes until you see that it is browning around the edges. Put the pan under the grill until the top has crisped up a bit and is a good deep brown.

If you want to top the mixture with eggs, half fill a medium non-stick saucepan with water, add a teaspoon of vinegar and bring it to the boil. And now for our special tip: place the eggs, still in their shells, into the boiling water for exactly 20 seconds – this helps the whites stay together. Remove them with a slotted spoon and turn the heat down so the water is simmering gently.

Crack the eggs into the water and cook for 3 minutes. The water should be gently bubbling and the eggs will rise to the surface when they are nearly ready. Remove them with a slotted spoon, drain briefly and place an egg on top of each helping of bubble and squeak.

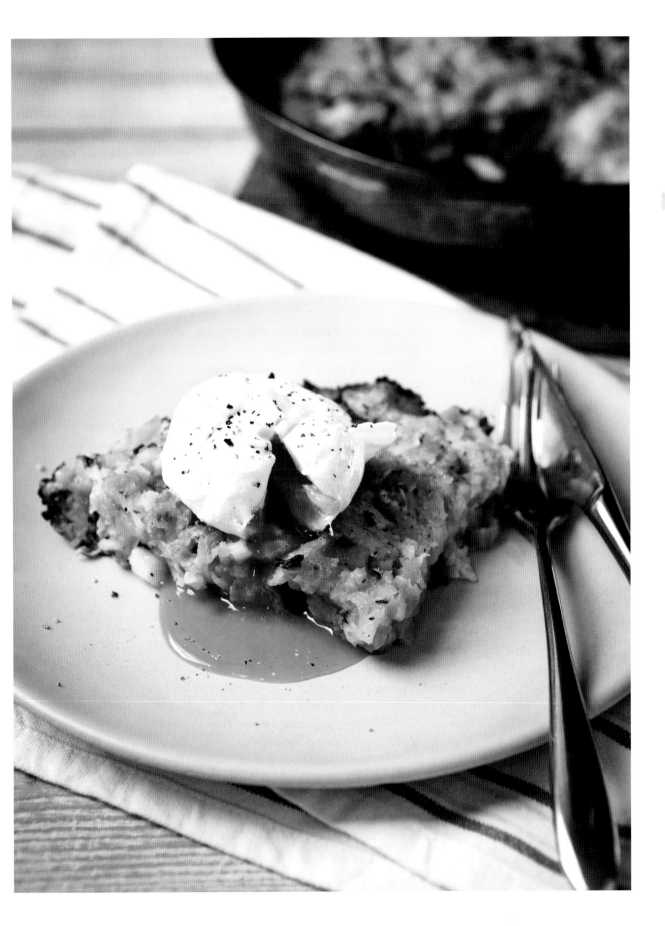

PASTA PUTTANESCA

250 calories per portion

This punchy pasta dish is a great store cupboard stand-by. It's so tasty you really don't need Parmesan as well. Up to you, but giving the cheese a miss does save on calories.

Serves 4
Prep: 8 minutes
Cooking time: 15–20 minutes

1 tsp olive oil
8 anchovy fillets
2 garlic cloves, finely chopped
1 red chilli, deseeded and finely
    chopped (or 1 tsp chilli flakes)
400g can of tomatoes or 4 large
    fresh tomatoes, peeled and
    chopped
100g pitted black olives, sliced
2 tbsp capers, rinsed
pinch of caster sugar (optional)
200g spaghetti
2 tbsp chopped parsley or basil
flaked sea salt
freshly ground black pepper

To make the sauce, heat the olive oil in a frying pan and add the anchovy fillets. Break them up with a wooden spoon, then add the garlic and chilli and fry for a couple of minutes before adding the tomatoes. Season with pepper – not salt at this stage. Simmer for about 15 minutes, then add the olives and capers and continue to simmer for a little longer – you want the sauce to be well reduced. Taste for seasoning and add salt if necessary. You might also want to add a pinch of caster sugar if the tomatoes are on the acidic side.

Meanwhile, bring a large saucepan of water to the boil and add salt. Drop in the spaghetti and cook until it is al dente. This should take 10–12 minutes, but check the packet instructions.

Drain the spaghetti and add it to the pan with the sauce. Mix thoroughly so the sauce coats all the spaghetti, then divide between bowls, making sure everyone gets plenty of sauce. Sprinkle with chopped parsley or basil and serve with a nice big green salad on the side.

FREEZE!

The sauce freezes well. To defrost, put it in a saucepan with a splash of water, then cover and heat gently until warmed through. Serve with freshly cooked pasta.

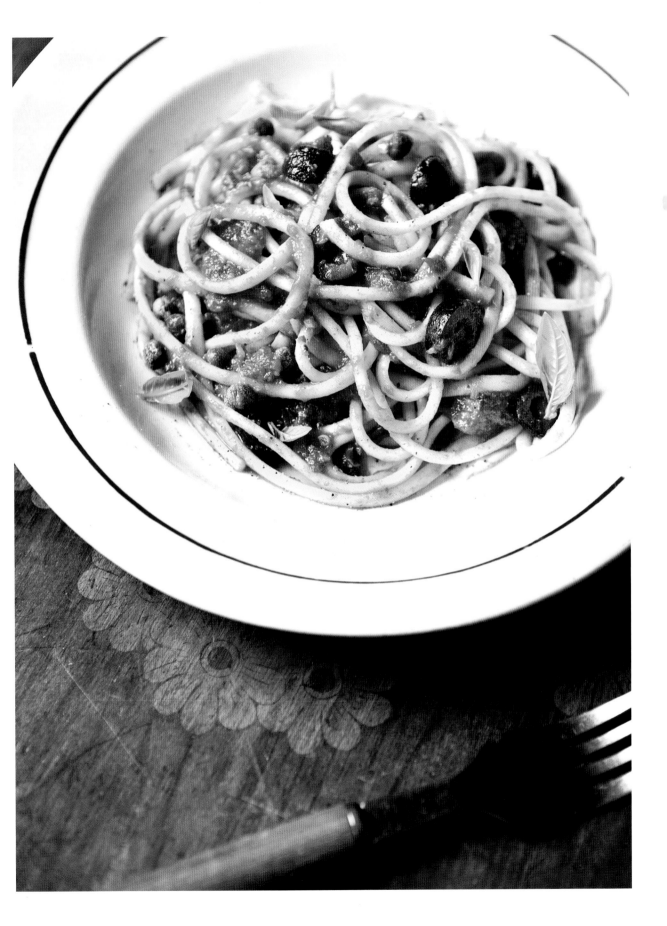

BAKED FISH WITH RED PEPPERS AND TOMATOES

200 calories per portion

This is a breeze to put together with some good cod, haddock or other fish and it's so good to eat. It's a great family supper but also good to serve when friends come over – let everyone open their own parcels at the table and enjoy the wafts of delicious saffrony, basily aromas. And it's so low cal that you can enjoy a few steamed new potatoes and green beans alongside.

Serves 4
Prep: 15 minutes
Cooking time: 20–25 minutes

1 tsp olive oil
1 red onion, sliced into thin wedges
2 red peppers, deseeded and sliced
    lengthways into strips
2 garlic cloves, finely chopped
1 mild red chilli, deseeded and
    finely chopped
100ml white wine
pinch of saffron threads
200g canned tomatoes (or fresh)
2 tbsp finely chopped parsley
2 tbsp finely chopped fresh basil
1 tsp grated lemon zest
oil, for spraying
4 thick fish fillets, about 150g each
4 thin slices of lemon
flaked sea salt
freshly ground black pepper

Preheat the oven to 200°C/Fan 180°C/Gas 6.

Heat the oil in a large non-stick frying pan. Add the onion and red peppers and fry them over a medium heat until they start to soften – you want them to stay fairly firm. Add the garlic and chilli and cook for another 2 minutes, stirring regularly.

Pour the white wine into the pan and crumble in the pinch of saffron. Simmer until most of the wine has evaporated, then add the tomatoes. Cook over a low heat for another 5 minutes, then stir in the parsley, basil and lemon zest.

Cut 4 large pieces of baking parchment or foil – they need to be big enough to make a parcel for each fish fillet. Spray each piece lightly with oil and place a fish fillet in the middle. Season with salt and pepper, then put a thin slice of lemon on top and add a quarter of the red pepper and tomato mixture to each parcel. Bring 2 opposite edges of the paper or foil together and fold them together. Fold over the remaining 2 edges to seal the parcel neatly. Wrap the remaining parcels in the same way.

Place the parcels on a baking tray and put them in the oven. Bake for 12–15 minutes, then open one slightly and check that the fish is cooked through. Take the parcels to the table so that everyone can open their own and enjoy the sensational scents.

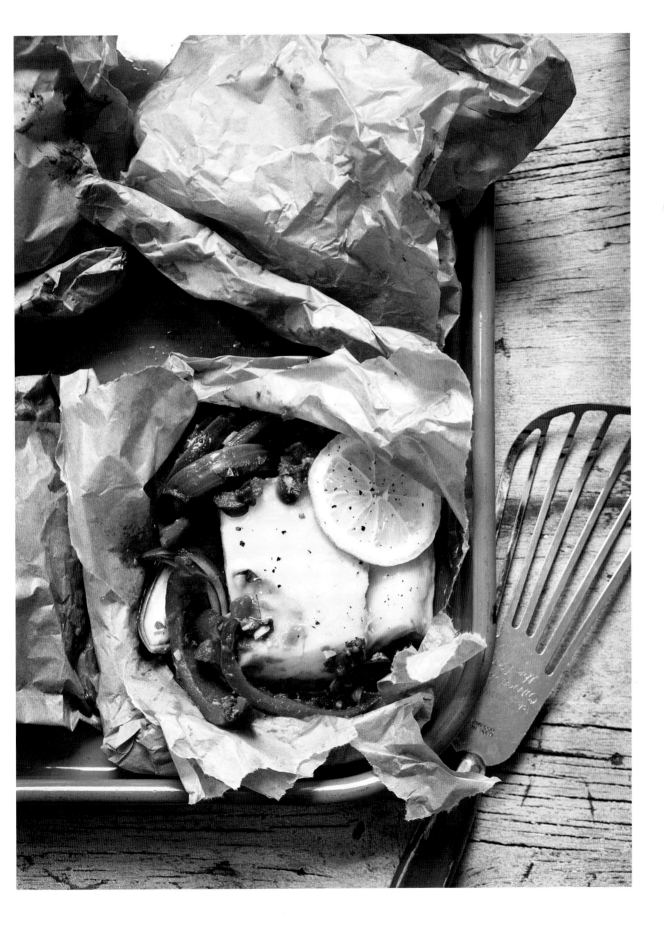

HOME-MADE FISH FINGERS

300 calories per portion

It's not only kids who love fish fingers! We do too and our home-made version beats the packet ones hands – or fingers – down. Spraying them with a bit of extra oil before cooking helps to give them a lovely golden colour and doesn't add many calories. We like these made with salmon but you can also use white fish, such as cod or haddock, which is lower in calories. And how about treating yourself to a fish finger wrap!

Serves 4
Prep: 10 minutes
Cooking time: 8–10 minutes

600g thick skinless salmon fillet
1 tbsp plain flour
1 tsp dried herbs (oregano or
  a mixture)
1 tsp finely grated lemon zest
4 tbsp low-fat natural yoghurt
50g fine breadcrumbs (such
  as Japanese panko)
oil, for spraying
flaked sea salt
freshly ground black pepper

Preheat the oven to 220°C/Fan 200°C/Gas 7. Line a baking tray with baking parchment.

Cut the fish fillets into 8 thick fingers. It's best to cut across the fillet if you can but don't worry if your fingers aren't perfectly even. Make sure they are completely dry by blotting with kitchen paper if necessary.

Mix the flour, herbs and grated lemon zest in a bowl and season with salt and pepper, then spread the mixture out on a plate. Spoon the yoghurt into a shallow bowl and spread the breadcrumbs on another plate.

Dip the fish fingers into the flour, shaking off any excess on to the plate. Then dip the flour-coated fish fingers into the yoghurt, again shaking off any excess, and lastly into the breadcrumbs, making sure they get a thorough coating.

Put the fish fingers on the lined baking tray and give them a light spray of oil – this isn't essential, but it will just help the colour along a little. Bake in the oven for 8–10 minutes, until they're starting to turn golden all over. Serve with some green veg or a salad and perhaps a dollop of ketchup – but don't forget to add 20 calories per spoonful!

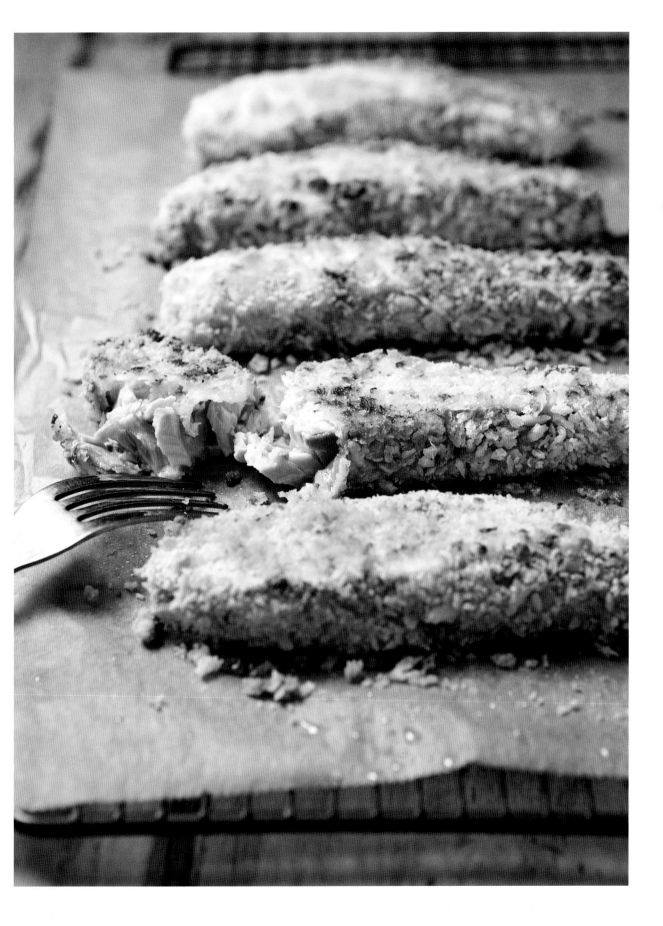

PRAWN AND TURKEY BALLS

312 calories per portion

You could use chicken for these cheeky little morsels, but turkey mince is readily available in supermarkets and slightly leaner than chicken. You'll see that the ingredients in the broth mirror those in the balls so everything in our Asian fantasia goes together beautifully. Clever eh? Remember that there are no calories in flavour so up the quantities of herbs and spices if you like.

Serves 4
Prep: 15 minutes
Cooking time: 15–20 minutes

250g raw prawns (shelled weight),
   roughly chopped
250g turkey mince
15g fresh root ginger, grated
2 garlic cloves, finely chopped
juice and grated zest of ½ a lime
a few coriander stems, chopped
1 tbsp fish sauce
50g breadcrumbs
flaked sea salt
freshly ground black pepper

Broth
400g can of reduced-fat
   coconut milk
200ml chicken stock
2 garlic cloves, finely chopped
15g fresh root ginger, chopped
1 shallot or half a small onion,
   finely sliced
2 tbsp chopped coriander stems
juice and grated zest of 1 lime
1 tbsp fish sauce
1 tsp sugar
1 red pepper, deseeded
   and cut into strips
100g baby corn
250g sprouting broccoli or pak choi
red chillies, sliced, to serve
coriander leaves, to serve

To make the prawn and turkey balls, put all the ingredients in a food processor and whizz them together to make a very smooth textured mixture. Leave the mixture to chill for half an hour and then, using damp hands, roll it into balls of about 35g each. You should end up with 16 balls. Chill the balls in the fridge until you are ready to cook them.

To make the broth, pour the coconut milk and chicken stock into a large wok or saucepan. Bring to the boil, then turn the heat down to a simmer and add the garlic, ginger, shallot, coriander stems, lime juice and zest, fish sauce and sugar. Allow the flavours to blend for a couple of minutes, then add the vegetables. Remove the balls from the fridge and add them to the broth, then simmer for about 10 minutes.

Check the broth for seasoning, then sprinkle over a couple of sliced chillies and some torn coriander leaves.

FREEZE!

You can freeze this as is, broth and all, but without the broccoli which will go soggy. Leave the broccoli out and add it to the broth when reheating.

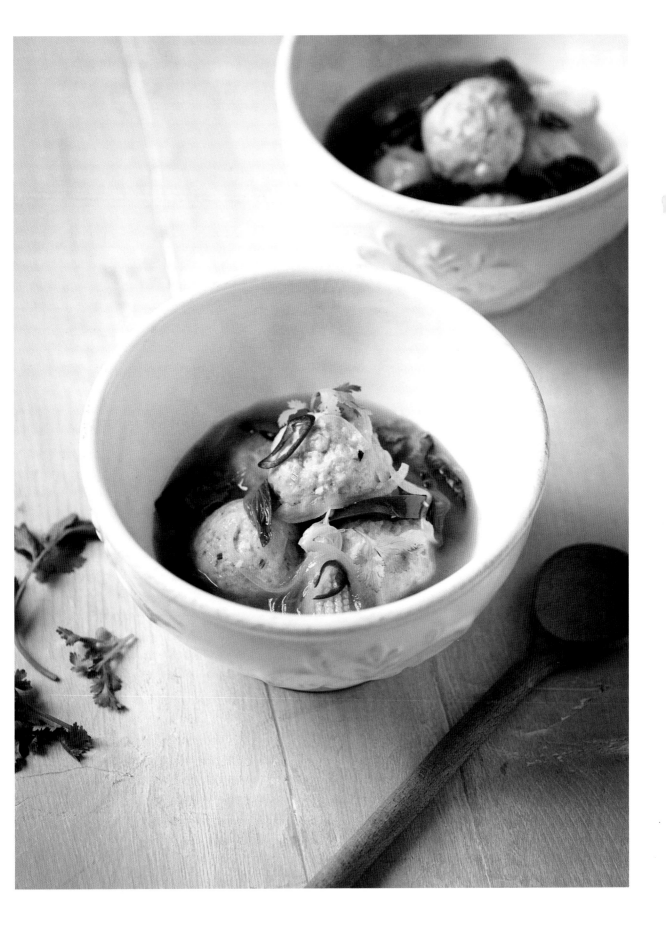

TRANSYLVANIAN MEATBALLS WITH GARLIC SAUCE

432 calories per portion (if serving 4); 288 calories per portion (if serving 6)

There's a double whammy of garlic in this indulgent recipe so it really keeps the vampires at bay! The meatballs cook beautifully in the oven and there's no need to brown them, as the paprika gives a lovely ochre colour. Great with a salad such as the fattoush on page 126.

Makes about 20 meatballs
Prep: 15 minutes
Cooking time: 20 minutes

1 tsp vegetable oil
1 onion, finely chopped
1 green pepper, deseeded
   and finely chopped
4 garlic cloves, finely chopped
600g lean beef mince
1 tbsp sweet paprika
100g breadcrumbs, Japanese panko
   are ideal
50g low-fat natural yoghurt
flaked sea salt
freshly ground black pepper

Garlic sauce
1 head of garlic, cloves separated
   but unpeeled
100g low-fat natural yoghurt
a pinch of caster sugar
1 tsp white wine vinegar

FREEZE!

The meatballs can be frozen raw or cooked, but don't freeze the sauce.

Preheat the oven to 220°C/Fan 200°C/Gas 7. Line a baking tray with baking parchment.

Heat the oil in a frying pan. Add the onion and green pepper and cook, stirring regularly, until the onion is soft and translucent. Add the garlic cloves and cook for another 2 minutes, then remove the pan from the heat and allow the veg to cool.

Put the beef in a large bowl and break it up. Season generously with salt and pepper and sprinkle over the paprika and breadcrumbs. Add the cooled onion, pepper and garlic, along with the yoghurt and mix the whole lot together. The easiest way to do this thoroughly is with your (very clean) hands.

Form the mixture into balls of about 40g each – the size of a golfball. Space them evenly on the baking tray and bake them in the oven for 12–15 minutes, until well browned.

Garlic sauce

To make the sauce, bring a small saucepan of water to the boil and add all the unpeeled garlic cloves. Simmer until the cloves are very tender – this should take about 15 minutes. Drain the garlic cloves and rinse them under cool running water until cool enough to handle. Squeeze the flesh out of the skins and then mash them on a chopping board with a fork.

Put the yoghurt in a bowl and add the mashed garlic, sugar and white wine vinegar. Season with salt and pepper and leave to stand for a few minutes before serving with the meatballs.

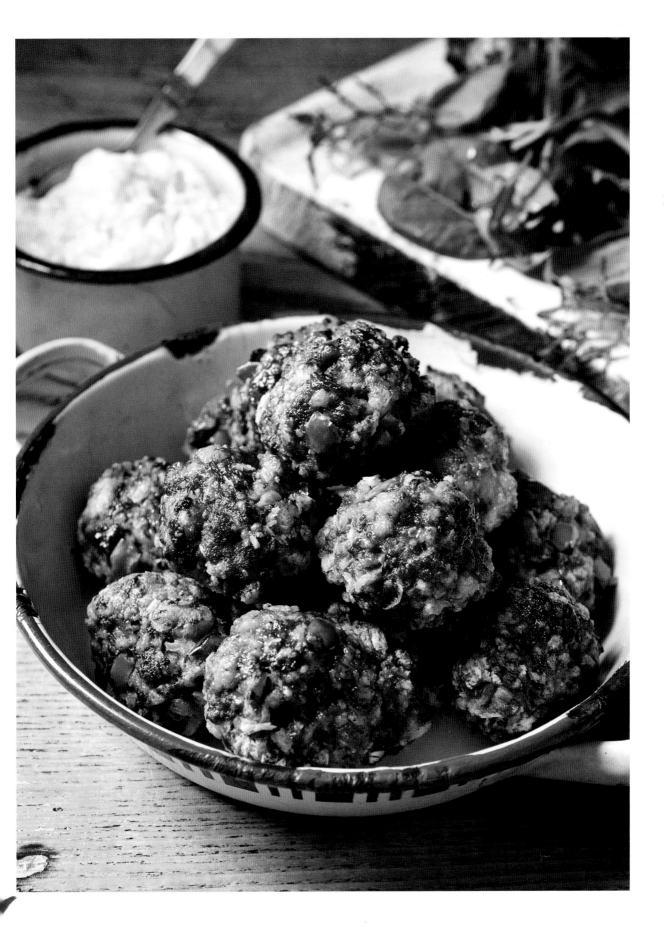

SMASHED-UP CHICKEN

316 calories per portion

You might recognise the title of this recipe from one of our earlier books. It makes a little chicken go a long way and was a great favourite but quite high-cal so we've tweaked and fiddled and got it down to a reasonable level for our new svelte selves. We've cut down on the fat content, reduced the amount of pasta a little, upped the veg and it still tastes the business.

Serves 4
Prep: 15 minutes
Cooking time: 25 minutes

---

4 skinless, boneless chicken thighs
1 tsp olive oil
200g button mushrooms, wiped
    and quartered
1 leek, trimmed and sliced into
    rounds
100ml white wine
125ml chicken stock
2 garlic cloves, crushed
1 tbsp fresh tarragon, finely
    chopped
1 tbsp lemon juice
freshly grated zest of 1 lemon
2 tbsp capers (rinsed and drained)
2 tbsp low-fat crème fraiche
handful of flatleaf parsley, chopped,
    to serve
flaked sea salt
freshly ground black pepper

Pasta
200g pasta (penne, fusilli –
    whatever you like)
1 tsp olive oil
1 tsp chilli flakes
1 garlic clove, crushed

Put a chicken thigh between 2 pieces of cling film and beat it with a rolling pin until thin. We really do want you to smash the chicken to bits, so don't be shy. Peel off the top layer of cling film and pull the chicken off in thin strips or ribbons. Repeat with the remaining thighs and season the chicken with salt and pepper.

Heat the oil in a non-stick frying pan. Cook the strips of chicken over a high heat until they are turning golden brown and just cooked through – this shouldn't take more than a couple of minutes, as the chicken strips are so thin. Take the chicken out of the pan and add the mushrooms. After a couple of minutes of cooking, they should start giving out some liquid. At this point, add the leek and sauté both together until the leek has started to soften.

Add the wine and stock to the pan and bring to the boil, stirring constantly to make sure nothing sticks to the bottom. Continue to cook to reduce the liquid and finish cooking the leek, then add the garlic, tarragon, lemon juice and zest. Cook for another 2 minutes, then add the capers.

Remove the pan from the heat and stir in the crème fraiche. Put the chicken back in the pan and warm it through again on a gentle heat. Check the seasoning.

Meanwhile, cook the pasta in plenty of salted, boiling water according to the packet instructions. Heat the olive oil in a separate pan, add the chilli flakes and garlic, then cook for just a minute. When the pasta is done, drain it well, then toss it in the chilli/garlic oil. Mix the chicken with the pasta and serve with plenty of chopped parsley sprinkled on top.

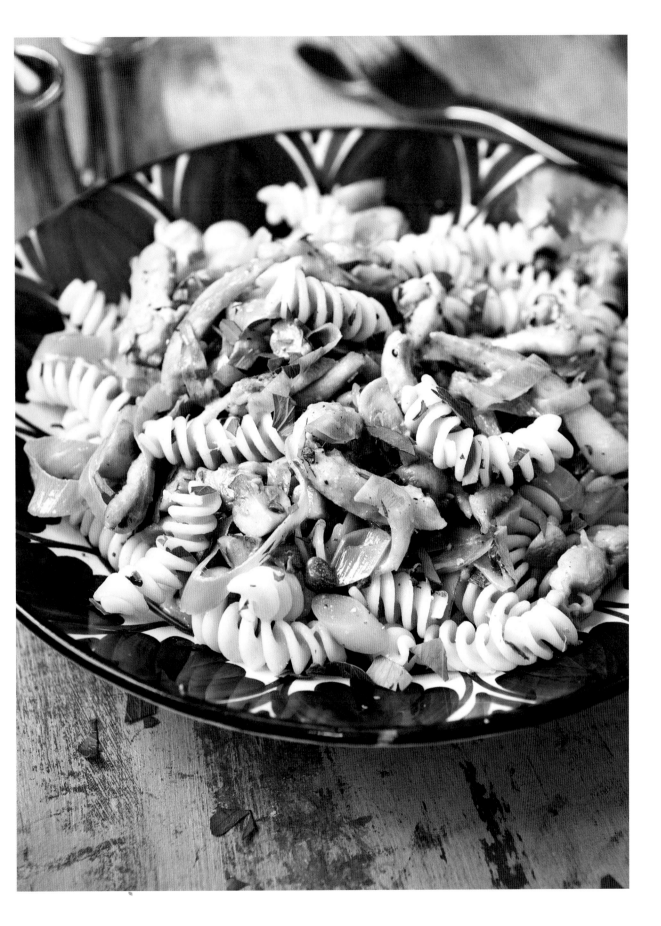

TURKEY CHILLI WITH CAULIFLOWER 'RICE'

300 calories per portion (with cauliflower); 240 calories (without cauliflower)

You can add a tiny bit of chocolate to this chilli which gives it a lovely rich mouth feel, but don't be tempted to eat the rest of the bar! Instead of serving the chilli with regular rice, try our cauliflower version, which tastes great and is very low calorie. Chipotle paste is available in supermarkets and delivers a real kick to the dish.

Serves 4
Prep: 15 minutes
Cooking time: 45 minutes

1 tsp vegetable oil
1 red onion, finely chopped
1 large red pepper, deseeded
    and diced
2 celery sticks, trimmed and diced
4 garlic cloves, finely chopped
500g turkey mince
1 tsp dried oregano
2 bay leaves
1 tbsp ground cumin
½ tsp ground allspice
1 tbsp chipotle paste
400g can of chopped tomatoes
400g can of beans (kidney, pinto,
    black-eyed peas), drained and
    rinsed
15g dark chocolate
flaked sea salt
freshly ground black pepper

To serve
fresh coriander leaves
lime wedges, for squeezing
low-fat crème fraiche

Cauliflower rice
1 cauliflower, broken up into florets
1 tsp cumin seeds
a small bunch of fresh coriander,
    chopped
flaked sea salt
freshly ground black pepper

Heat the oil in a large saucepan, then add the onion, pepper and celery. Cook over a low heat for 5 minutes, until the veg are starting to soften, then add the garlic and the turkey mince. Turn up the heat slightly and cook until the turkey has browned all over. Keep stirring and use the spoon to break up any clumps of turkey mince.

Add the oregano, bay leaves, cumin, allspice and chipotle paste. Give everything a good stir so it all gets coated with the paste, then pour in the chopped tomatoes and 250ml water. Add the drained beans and season with salt and pepper.

Bring to the boil, then cover the pan and simmer the chilli over a low heat for half an hour, until the sauce has thickened. Keep an eye on it and add a drop more water towards the end if you think it is in danger of catching. Five minutes from the end of the cooking time, add the chocolate. To serve, divide between 4 plates, sprinkle with coriander leaves and add a wedge of lime and a dessertspoon of crème fraiche to each serving.

Cauliflower rice
Break the cauliflower up into florets. Put these in a food processor and blitz until the cauliflower has the texture of large breadcrumbs.

Heat a non-stick frying pan and dry-fry the cumin seeds for a few moments until they start to give off a spicy aroma. Coat the bottom of the pan with water – about 100ml should do it. Evenly spread the cauliflower crumbs over the frying pan and season. Cook over a medium heat for about 5 minutes, stirring fairly regularly until the water has evaporated and the cauliflower is looking quite dry. Stir in the coriander and remove the pan from the heat. Fork the cauliflower over and it will 'fluff up' nicely.

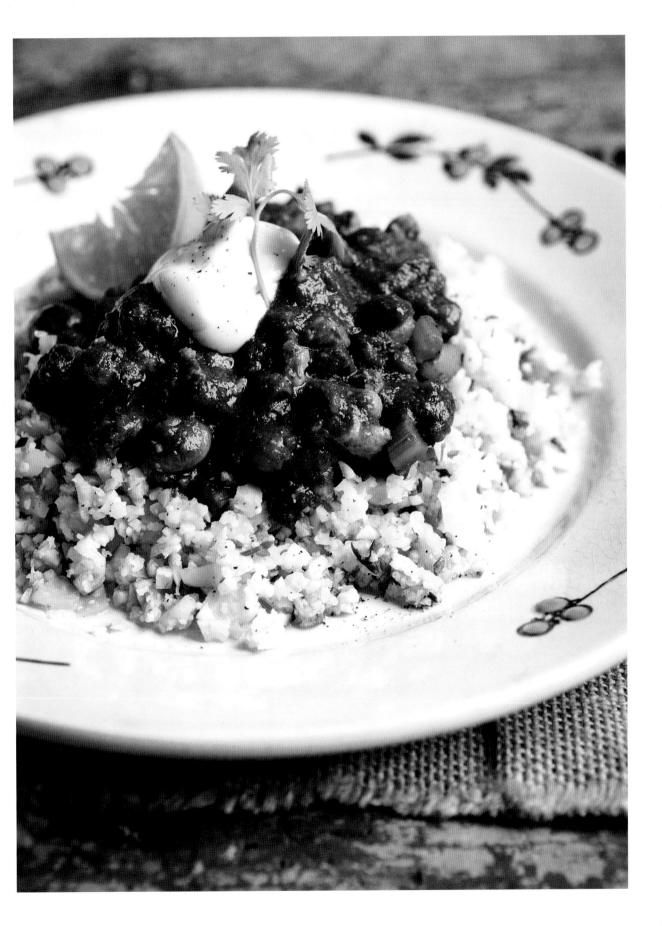

CHICKEN WITH CITRUS RUB AND BRAISED LENTILS

chicken: 166 calories per portion; chicken and lentils: 400 calories per portion

Slicing the chicken through the middle into thin pieces means it cooks really quickly and stays tender. The citrus rub adds bags of flavour and is so easy to do. This recipe makes plenty of rub mixture but it keeps well for another time. It's best to get unwaxed fruit if you can, but otherwise give the lemons and oranges a good scrub in hot water to melt off the wax. The chicken is great with the braised lentils but also good with the Greek roast veg on page 134.

Serves 4
Prep: 25 minutes
Cooking time: 1 hour 45 minutes

4 skinless, boneless chicken breasts
1 tsp olive oil

Rub
finely grated zest of 2 oranges
finely grated zest of 1 lemon
2 long sprigs of rosemary
10g black peppercorns
25g coarse salt

Braised lentils
1 tsp olive oil
1 onion, finely chopped
2 celery sticks, trimmed and diced
2 carrots, peeled and diced
100g mushrooms, wiped clean
  and finely chopped
2 garlic cloves, finely chopped
a few sprigs of thyme
1 tsp sage
150g puy lentils (or green or
  brown lentils)
75ml white wine
600ml chicken stock or water
1 tbsp tomato purée
2 tbsp finely chopped parsley
flaked sea salt
freshly ground black pepper

First make the rub. Preheat the oven to its lowest setting and line a tray with baking parchment. Spread the zest and rosemary over the baking tray. Put the tray in the oven for half an hour, then remove and break up any clumps of zest. Put the tray back in the oven for another hour, adding the peppercorns for the last 10 minutes. Remove from the oven and allow the mixture to cool. Tip it all into a spice grinder with the salt and whizz until you have a fairly fine powder. Decant the powder into a jar – it will keep indefinitely.

Now for the chicken. Using a sharp knife, cut into the middle of the breast and continue slicing until you have cut the breast into 2 thin pieces. Put a slice between 2 pieces of cling film and flatten with a meat hammer or rolling pin until it is about 5mm thick. Repeat with the remaining breasts.

Dust the rub all over the chicken. You won't need much – perhaps half a teaspoon per piece. Heat the oil in a large frying pan. Add a few pieces of chicken and cook on one side for 2 minutes or until they are a deep golden brown, then flip them over and cook on the other side for 2–3 minutes. Check whether the chicken is done – if it isn't, cook for another minute or so. The exact time will depend on the thickness of your chicken but make sure that no pinkness remains. Keep the chicken warm while you cook the rest.

Braised lentils
Heat the oil in a large saucepan. Add the onion, celery, carrots and mushrooms to the pan and cook, stirring regularly, over a medium heat until the veg are starting to brown round the edges. Add the garlic and cook for another 2 minutes, then add the thyme and sage.

Rinse the puy lentils well and add them to the saucepan. Pour over the wine and stock and season with salt and pepper. Bring the mixture to the boil and cover the pan with a lid. Simmer for 15 minutes, then add the tomato purée.

Simmer uncovered for another 15 minutes until the lentils are tender, stirring regularly to check that there is enough liquid in the pan. If you think the lentils are in danger of sticking, add a little more water or stock. Sprinkle with parsley before serving.

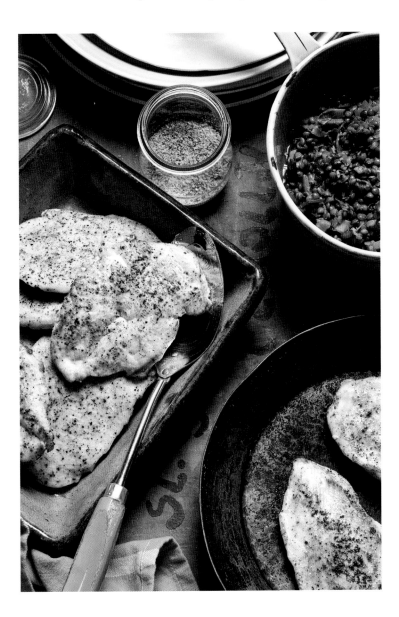

FRIDAY NIGHT SUPPERS

It's Friday night, you're looking forward to the weekend and you feel like a treat, but you don't want to undo all your good work. Fear not – there's no need to be tempted by the local kebab shop when you can try some of our mouth-watering versions of dishes like samosas, beef curry and stir-fries. And you won't believe our special fusion tandoori chicken, coated with a mix of curry paste, dill and capers. Sounds bonkers but it's a taste sensation.

PRAWN STIR-FRY WITH COURGETTE 'NOODLES'

180 calories per portion

We were dead chuffed with the lasagne we made using pieces of leek instead of pasta in our first Hairy Dieters' book, so we thought we'd try making noodles with strips of courgette! They're fab and ridiculously low calorie. Be warned – when you prepare the courgettes they will look like a huge heap but they do wilt down a lot so don't worry. There's a lovely little Thai lilt to this dish and we're sure you'll enjoy it.

Serves 4
Prep: 20 minutes
Cooking time: 8–10 minutes

400g large peeled raw tiger prawns,
    deveined if necessary
1 small bunch of coriander leaves,
    stems and leaves separated
2 large courgettes
1 tbsp vegetable oil
1 onion, sliced into thin wedges
1 red pepper, sliced into strips
1 carrot, cut into matchsticks
100g green beans, cut in half
100g baby corn, sliced in half
    lengthways
1 tbsp soy sauce
225g can of bamboo shoots,
    drained
100g bean sprouts

Marinade
2 garlic cloves, crushed
1 small red chilli, deseeded and
    finely chopped
1 lemon grass stalk, finely sliced
freshly squeezed juice and finely
    grated zest of 1 lime
10g chunk of fresh root ginger,
    peeled and grated
2 tbsp fish sauce
1 tsp caster sugar

Put the prawns in a bowl. Put all the marinade ingredients and the coriander stems in a food processor or blender and blitz until well combined – the mixture doesn't have to be very smooth. Pour this over the prawns and stir well so they are all coated. Set aside while you prepare the vegetables.

Top and tail the courgettes. Using a vegetable peeler, cut them into long strips, making them as thin as you can. Cut these strips in half lengthways until you have a large pile of noodle-like ribbons of courgette, each about 1cm wide.

Heat the oil in a wok or large frying pan until it's at smoking point and add the onion, red pepper and carrot. Cook over a very high heat for 2 minutes, stirring constantly, then add the green beans and baby corn. Continue to cook over a very high heat for another couple of minutes, then add the soy sauce. Finally, add the bamboo shoots, bean sprouts and courgettes. Turn everything over for a minute until the courgette noodles start to wilt. Be careful here – if you cook them for too long they will start to collapse and give out too much water. You want them to stay nice and firm.

Divide the vegetables between your serving plates, then immediately throw the prawns, with their marinade, into the wok. Stir over a high heat until the prawns are just cooked through and starting to char slightly. Add the prawns to the vegetables and serve immediately with the coriander leaves sprinkled over.

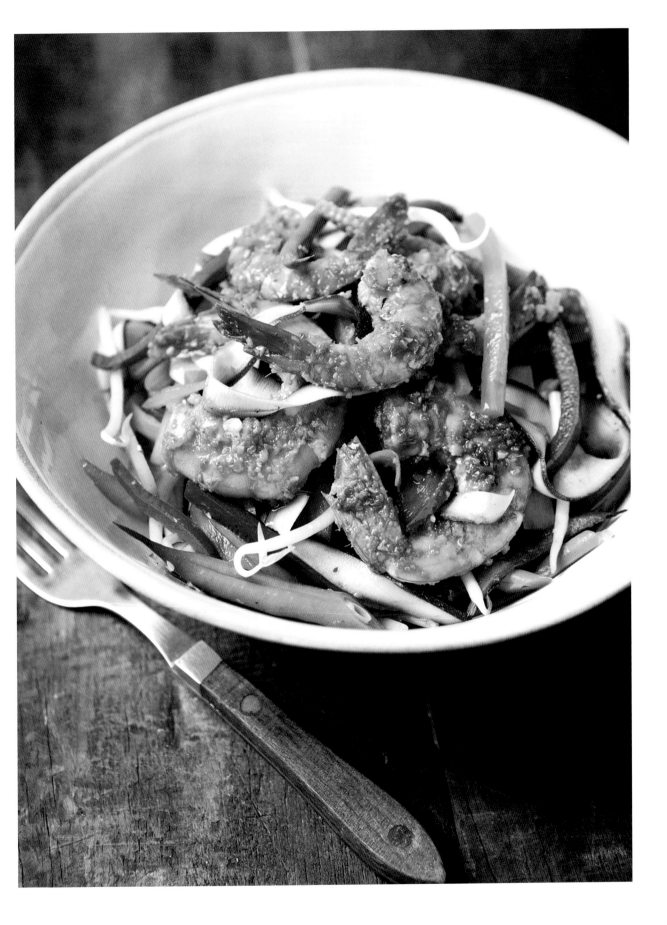

SAMOSAS

71 calories per meat samosa; 65 calories per veggie samosa

Over the years we've come up with a number of samosa recipes – they're a guilty pleasure we don't want to give up. These work a treat and we've found that you can bake them in the oven instead of deep-frying, so saving lots of calories.

Makes 18
Prep: 30–45 minutes
Cooking time: 30–45 minutes

6 sheets of filo pastry
oil, for spraying

Meat filling
1 tbsp vegetable oil
175g lean chicken or turkey mince
1 onion, finely chopped
50g butternut squash, peeled and
    finely diced
2 garlic cloves, finely chopped
5g chunk of fresh root ginger,
    peeled and finely chopped
1 tsp garam masala
1 tsp nigella seeds
½ tsp turmeric
50g peas (fresh or frozen)
squeeze of lemon juice
2 tbsp finely chopped coriander
    leaves
flaked sea salt
freshly ground black pepper

To make the meat filling, heat the oil in a non-stick frying pan and add the mince and onion. Cook for 5 minutes until the meat is cooked through and the onion has softened. Add the squash, garlic and ginger and cook for another 2 minutes. Add the garam masala, nigella seeds and turmeric, then pour in 100ml of water. Add the peas and season with salt and pepper. Simmer over a gentle heat until the squash is tender and most of the liquid has evaporated. Add a squeeze of lemon juice, then stir in the chopped coriander. Leave the filling to cool at least to room temperature before you start assembling the samosas.

To make the vegetable filling, heat the oil in a non-stick frying pan. Add the onion and potato and cook, stirring regularly, for 5 minutes until soft. Proceed with the remaining ingredients exactly as for the meat filling and leave to cool.

To make the shells for the samosas, lay out a sheet of filo. Cut out rounds measuring about 16cm in diameter. You should be able to get 3 rounds from each sheet. You can make a template out of cardboard for this, or find a plate or bowl that is about the right size.

Fold a round in half to make a semi-circle and place it with the straight side at the bottom. Take the outer right corner and fold the pastry over so it overlaps half of the rest of the semicircle of pastry. Take the outer left corner and fold it over the rest of the pastry to make a cone shape. Wet the outside edges and press to make sure they are securely stuck to the rest of the pastry.

Open up the cone and make sure there are 3 layers of pastry on each side. Add about a dessertspoon of filling – do this a teaspoon at a time so you can get more filling into the bottom corner of the cone. Make sure you leave a border around the top of at least half a centimetre. Fold one side of the border down on top of the filling, then dampen each of the 3 layers of remaining border and fold this over to close the samosa. Make sure there are no loose edges and pinch each of the 3 corners. Repeat to use all the filo and stuffing.

When you are almost ready to bake the samosas, preheat the oven to 220°C/Fan 200°C/Gas 7. Place the samosas on a baking tray and spray them lightly with oil. Bake in the preheated oven for 15–20 minutes until crisp and golden brown in patches.

Vegetable filling

1 tbsp vegetable oil
1 onion, finely chopped
200g potato, finely diced
2 garlic cloves, finely chopped
5g chunk of fresh root ginger, peeled and finely chopped
1 tsp garam masala
1 tsp nigella seeds
½ tsp turmeric
50g peas (fresh or frozen)
squeeze of lemon juice
2 tbsp finely chopped coriander leaves
flaked sea salt
freshly ground black pepper

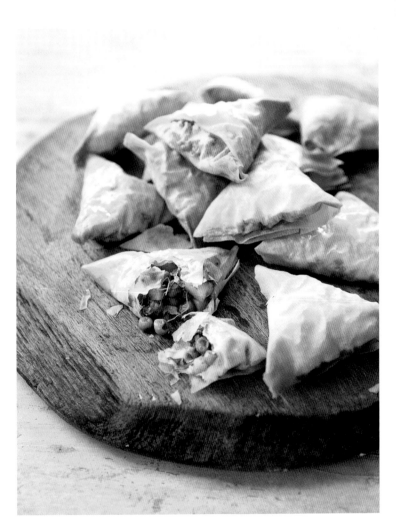

FREEZE!

Samosas are probably best frozen once assembled but uncooked. The bonus is that unlike deep-fried samosas, these seem to stay beautifully crisp and light even when they've cooled down. While you're at it you could make double the quantity.

LAMB DHANSAK

336 calories per portion

This is a proper curry and we've trimmed the calories while keeping it punchy and delicious. Although we love curry pastes, we've discovered that they're higher in calories than powder.

Serves 6
Prep: 20 minutes
Cooking time: 2 hours 15 minutes

1 tbsp vegetable oil
2 large onions, thinly sliced
750g lean lamb leg meat, diced
20g chunk of fresh root ginger, peeled and grated
4 garlic cloves, finely chopped
3 green chillies, deseeded and finely chopped
2 tbsp medium curry powder
1 tbsp ground cumin
1 tbsp ground coriander
1 tsp turmeric
2 bay leaves
150g red lentils
½ butternut squash, cut into large chunks
juice of 1 lime
handful of chopped coriander leaves, to garnish
flaked sea salt
freshly ground black pepper

Heat the oil in a large casserole dish or heavy-based saucepan. Add the onions and cook over a low heat until they have softened but not browned. This should take about 15 minutes. Turn up the heat slightly and add the lamb, ginger, garlic and chillies. Sprinkle all the spices over the meat and season with salt and pepper. Stir for a couple of minutes until the lamb is well coated with spices.

Add the bay leaves and the red lentils, then pour in 700ml water. Slowly bring to the boil, turn the heat down and leave to simmer for an hour. Add the butternut squash and cook for another half an hour, then remove the lid and leave the curry to simmer, uncovered, for another 15 minutes.

Check the seasoning, add the lime juice and sprinkle with chopped coriander before serving. Lovely served with some cauliflower rice (see page 48).

FREEZE!

This freezes well. The flavours of the ginger and garlic will intensify on freezing, but in a good way. Just be careful when defrosting and reheating not to stir too much, as cooked, frozen lamb has a tendency to shred. To avoid soggy butternut squash, prepare the dish up to the point that the butternut squash is added, then freeze and add the squash when reheating.

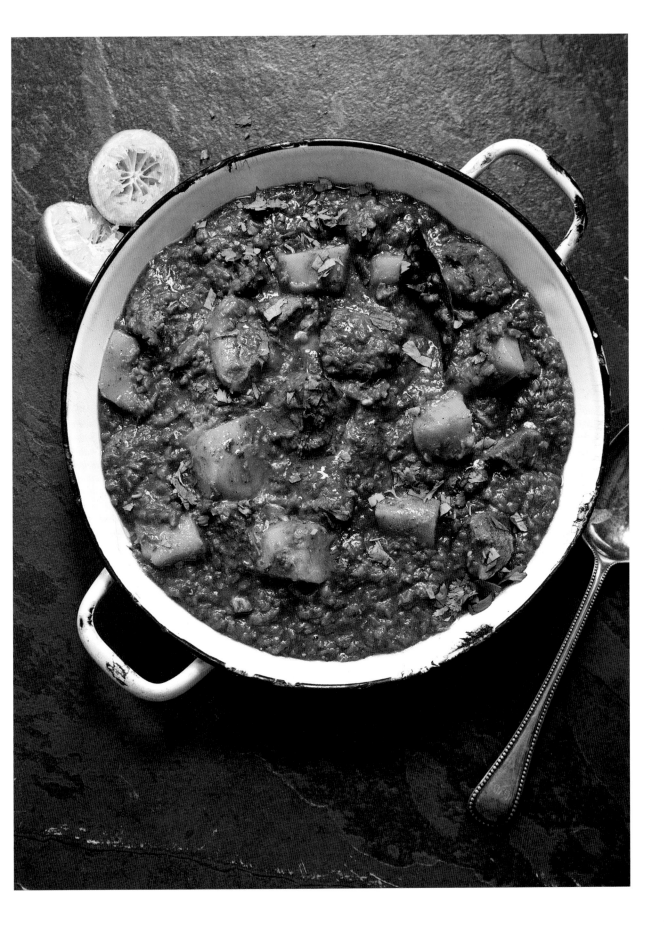

VEGETABLE CURRY

91 calories per portion

There's more fibre in this veggie treat than a brillo pad and it's much tastier of course! Vegetable curries, especially those with aubergine, often contain lots of oil. We've kept the oil as low as possible in this by cooking the aubergine on a fairly high heat so it seals quickly and doesn't soak up too much. The mushrooms also give out some liquid, which helps keep things nice and juicy. Serve with rice for a veggie main meal or as an accompaniment to a meat dish.

Serves 4
Prep: 15 minutes
Cooking time: 30–35 minutes

1 tbsp vegetable oil
1 tsp cumin seeds
1 onion, thickly sliced
1 aubergine, diced
200g mushrooms, wiped
  and halved
1 courgette, diced
2 garlic cloves, finely chopped
10g chunk of fresh root ginger,
  peeled and grated
1 tbsp medium curry powder
100g green beans, halved
400g can of tomatoes
large handful of fresh coriander
  leaves
flaked sea salt
freshly ground black pepper

To serve
4 tbsp fat-free natural yoghurt
1 tsp dried mint (optional)

Heat the oil in a large frying pan and add the cumin seeds, onion, aubergine, mushrooms and courgette. Cook over a medium heat, stirring regularly, until the vegetables have started to soften around the edges and have taken on a bit of colour.

Add the garlic and ginger, then sprinkle over the curry powder and season with salt and pepper. Add the green beans and pour in 200ml of water. Simmer for 2 minutes, then add the tomatoes. Simmer for about 20 minutes, until the vegetables are tender and the curry has thickened.

Just before serving, stir in a large handful of fresh coriander. Serve with yoghurt – stir some dried mint into it if you like.

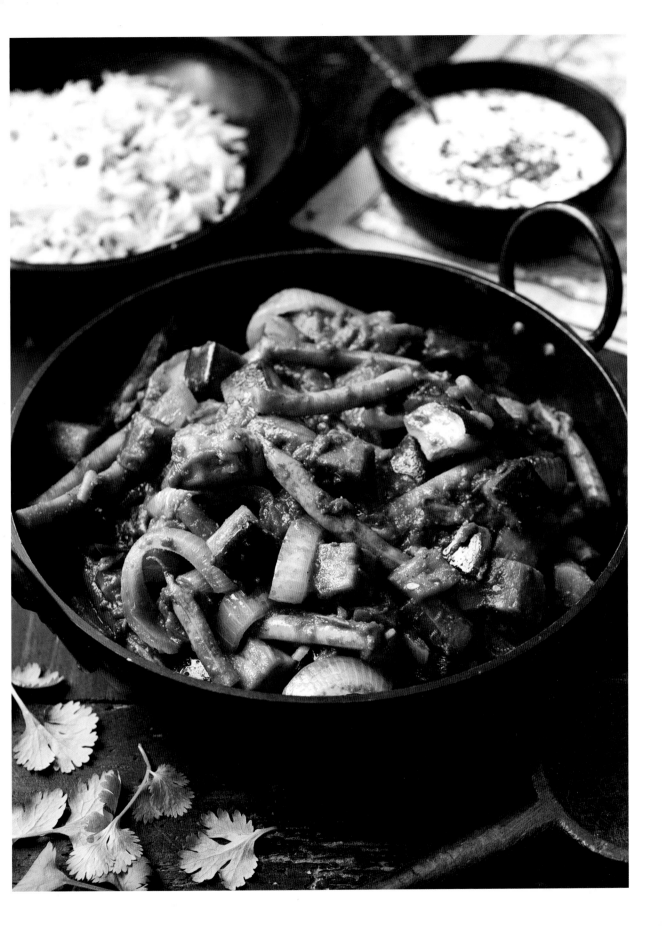

PIZZAS WITH 3 TOPPINGS

*420 calories per meat feast pizza; 322 calories per Parma ham, courgette
and mushroom pizza; 405 calories per spinach and egg pizza*

*The dough recipe will make 4 very thin pizzas of about 20cm in diameter. Don't worry if they're
not perfectly round – they look more rustic and taste just as good. Each topping recipe makes
enough for four pizzas and the mozzarella is divided between them. Top tip: if you've made
our turkey chilli on page 48 and you've got some left over, it makes a brilliant pizza topping!*

Serves 4
Prep: 15 minutes, plus 1 hour
rising time
Cooking time: 26–40 minutes

Pizza dough
250g strong white flour
5g dried yeast
½ tsp salt
150ml tepid water

Tomato sauce
400g can of tomatoes
2 garlic cloves
1 tsp dried oregano
large handful of basil, shredded
flaked sea salt
freshly ground black pepper

1 ball of half-fat mozzarella, very
    thinly sliced

Meat feast
1 tsp olive oil
1 onion, finely chopped
200g lean beef mince
1 tsp ground cumin
1 tsp ground coriander
2 tbsp sliced jalapeño chillies
1 red pepper, deseeded and sliced
    thinly into rounds

To make the pizza dough, mix the flour, yeast and salt, then gradually
add the water until you have a dough. Either turn the dough out on
to a floured work surface and knead until smooth and elastic (about
5 minutes) or knead with the dough hook in a food mixer. Put the
dough in a bowl and cover with a damp tea towel. Leave until it has
doubled in size – this will probably take about an hour. Knock it
back and cut it into 4 pieces – best to do this by weight.

To make the sauce, put the tomatoes, garlic and oregano in a saucepan
and season with salt and pepper. Simmer until the tomatoes have
reduced to a thick paste – 20–30 minutes. Add the basil, then blitz with
a blender until smooth.

Preheat your oven to its highest setting and heat a couple of upturned
baking trays. Roll each ball of dough out into a round of about
20cm in diameter. Put a couple of spoonfuls of sauce on each base
and spread it over evenly. Add 3–4 slices of mozzarella to each pizza,
then finish with your chosen topping (see below). Slide the pizzas on
to the hot baking trays – you should be able to get 2 on each. Bake
for about 6 minutes.

Meat feast topping

Heat the oil in a frying pan and add the onion. Fry over a
medium heat until the onion has softened and is starting to
go brown, as this will add sweetness. Add the beef, then sprinkle
over the spices. Season with salt and pepper and fry until the beef
is just cooked through. Divide this mixture between the pizzas and
top with the jalepeños and red pepper.

Parma ham, courgette and mushroom topping

Sprinkle the grated courgette and the sliced mushrooms over the tomato sauce on the pizzas. Tear up each slice of Parma ham and arrange it on top and sprinkle over the herbs.

Spinach and egg topping

Wash the spinach thoroughly, then without draining it too thoroughly, put it in a saucepan and cook until it has wilted down completely. Wait until it is cool enough to handle, then squeeze out as much of the moisture as you can. Season with salt, a grating of nutmeg and the lemon zest. Divide the spinach between the 4 pizzas. The best way to arrange it is in a circular 'wall', large enough to contain the egg. Break an egg on to each pizza and sprinkle over the Parmesan cheese.

Parma ham with courgettes and mushrooms
½ courgette, grated
8 mushrooms, wiped and thinly sliced
4 slices of Parma ham
a few sprigs of thyme
basil leaves, roughly torn

Spinach and egg
200g fresh spinach
a grating of nutmeg
1 tsp finely grated lemon zest
4 eggs
10g Parmesan cheese, finely grated

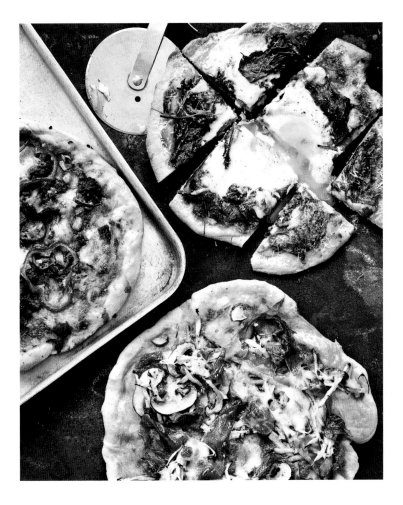

SWEDISH MEATBALLS

473 calories per portion (if serving 4); 315 calories per portion (if serving 6)

These will bring back memories of the meatballs served at a certain Scandinavian megastore but they are really easy to make at home. Stick some Abba on and enjoy our Swedish supper – you'll be living the dream!

Serves 4–6 (makes about
24 meatballs)
Prep: 20 minutes
Cooking time: 40 minutes

1 tbsp olive oil
1 onion, finely chopped
1 garlic clove, finely chopped
300g lean beef mince
300g lean pork mince
1 tbsp anchovy paste
100g breadcrumbs
50ml milk
½ tsp allspice
¼ tsp nutmeg
1 tsp flaked sea salt
freshly ground black pepper
a few sprigs of dill, to serve

Gravy
100ml white wine
500ml well-flavoured beef stock
2 tbsp single cream
1 tbsp lingonberry jam, melted and
  sieved if you want to get rid of
  the fruit (or redcurrant
  or cranberry jelly)
up to 1 tbsp arrowroot
flaked sea salt
freshly ground black pepper

Preheat the oven to 200°C/Fan 180°C/Gas 6. To make the meatballs, heat the oil in a frying pan and cook the onion until it's soft and translucent. Add the garlic and cook for another minute. Remove the pan from the heat and allow the onion and garlic to cool.

Put all the meatball ingredients, including the onion and garlic, into a large bowl and mix thoroughly with your hands. Shape the mixture into balls between the size of a walnut and a golf ball – they should be about 40g in weight. Put the balls on a baking tray and bake for 12–15 minutes until cooked through.

To make the gravy, put the wine in a saucepan and boil fiercely until it has reduced by about half – this is to cook most of the alcohol taste out of it. Add the stock and simmer for 5 minutes, then stir in the single cream and the jam. Season with salt and pepper. Mix the arrowroot with a little water and add a teaspoon of the mixture at a time to the gravy, stirring thoroughly and simmering briefly between each addition until it has started to thicken.

Put the meatballs in the gravy and simmer for another 5 minutes to allow all the flavours to combine – this is important for the taste of the gravy so don't be tempted to skip this stage. Serve with a sprinkling of dill.

FREEZE!

The cooked meatballs freeze well. Open freeze them on a tray, then pop them into freezer bags or a plastic box once they're solid. The gravy is best made fresh. Gently reheat the defrosted meatballs in the gravy before serving.

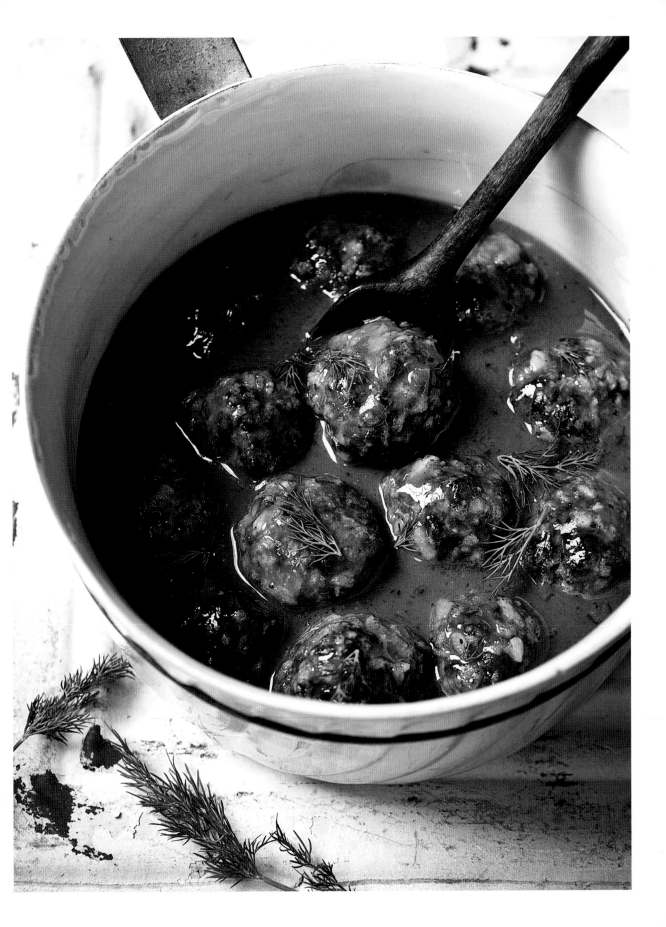

LEMON CHICKEN

186 calories per portion

Great served with plain rice and some Chinese greens or steamed pak choi. The trick with the egg white is called velveting and gives an authentic Chinese texture to the chicken.

Serves 4
Prep: 10 minutes, plus 20 minutes chilling
Cooking time: 10–12 minutes

4 fairly small chicken breasts
    (about 100–150g each) sliced
    into strips
1 egg white
2 tsp cornflour
1 tbsp vegetable oil
2 spring onions, sliced, to serve

Sauce
100ml chicken stock
juice of 2 lemons
1 tsp caster sugar
1 tbsp light soy sauce
1 tbsp rice wine (mirin)
3 garlic cloves
½ tsp chilli flakes
½ tsp cornflour
a few drops of sesame oil
flaked sea salt
freshly ground black pepper

Put the chicken strips in a bowl. Whisk together the egg white and cornflour, making as smooth a paste as you can. Pour this over the chicken and mix thoroughly so the chicken is completely coated. Chill for 20 minutes in the fridge.

Heat the oil in a wok until it starts to smoke then add all the chicken. Toss the chicken around the wok until it is golden brown and completely cooked through, with no sign of pinkness. This shouldn't take longer than a couple of minutes. Remove the chicken from wok and set aside.

To make the sauce, put the wok back on the hob but over a lower heat. Add the chicken stock, lemon juice, sugar, soy sauce, rice wine, garlic cloves and chilli flakes and season well with salt and pepper. Bring to the boil, then turn the heat down and simmer for a minute.

Mix the cornflour with a small amount of water until you have a smooth, thin paste. Pour this into the sauce and simmer until the sauce has thickened slightly. Put the chicken back in the wok and simmer until it has warmed through again. Finally, add a few drops of sesame oil.

Let the whole thing sit for a few minutes to allow the flavours to develop – this is important for the final taste of the sauce. Sprinkle with the sliced spring onions before serving.

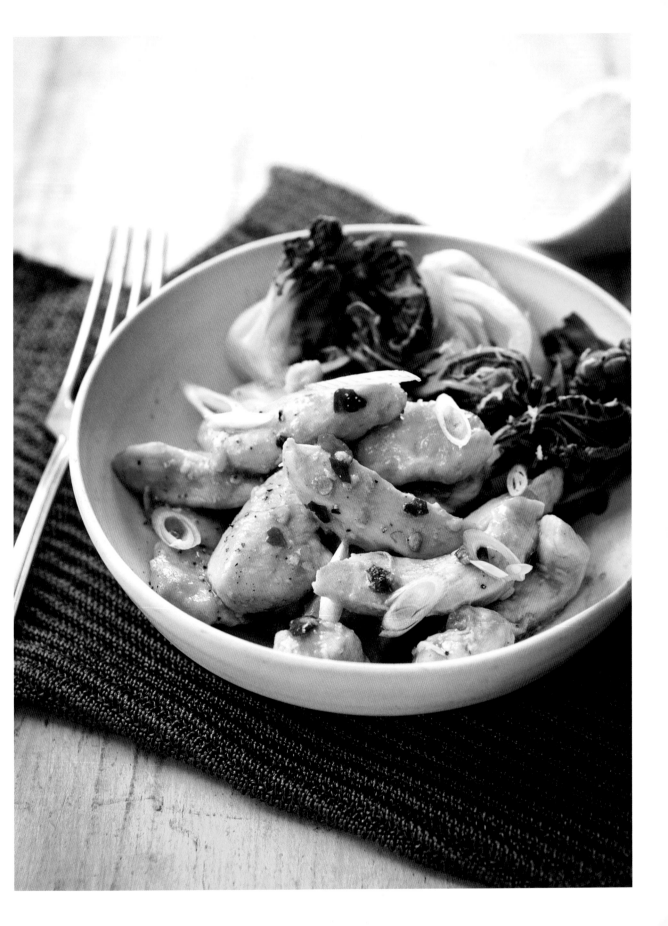

CARIBBEAN CHICKEN CURRY

290 calories per portion

This is a proper carnival of a dish and has everything you need in one scrumptious pot full of Caribbean flavours. You can buy Caribbean curry powder in most supermarkets.

Serves 4
Prep: 20 minutes
Cooking time: 1 hour 30 minutes

8 bone-in chicken thighs,
   skinned and trimmed of fat
1½ limes
1 tbsp vegetable oil
300ml chicken stock or water
1 large sprig of thyme
2 bay leaves
200g piece of pumpkin, peeled
   and cut into large chunks
1 large potato, peeled and cut
   into large chunks
100g pineapple, diced
1 tsp rum (optional)
2 spring onions, finely sliced
2 tbsp chopped flatleaf parsley
flaked sea salt
freshly ground black pepper

Curry paste
1 onion, roughly chopped
4 garlic cloves, peeled and cut
   in half
15g chunk of fresh root ginger,
   peeled and roughly chopped
2 scotch bonnet chillies (or to
   taste), deseeded and finely
   chopped
2 tbsp medium curry powder,
   preferably Caribbean
½ tsp ground allspice

Put the chicken thighs in a bowl and add the juice of 1 lime and about 100ml of water. Rub the lime juice over the chicken and leave for a few minutes while you make the paste.

For the paste, put the onion, garlic, ginger, scotch bonnets, curry powder and ground allspice in a food processor or blender and add a tablespoon of water. Blitz until fairly smooth.

Heat the vegetable oil in a large casserole dish over a medium heat. Add the paste and cook, stirring constantly, for a couple of minutes. Now add the chicken and season with salt and pepper. Stir so the chicken is coated with the paste, then pour in 300ml of chicken stock or water and add the thyme and bay leaves.

Bring the mixture to the boil, then turn down the heat to a gentle simmer and cover. Cook for about 45 minutes, then add the pumpkin, potato and pineapple. Cook for another 30 minutes, covered, then take off the lid. Add the juice of the remaining half a lime and, if you like, a teaspoon of rum, then cook, uncovered, for another 10 minutes to allow the sauce to reduce a little. Sprinkle the spring onions and parsley over the top of the curry and serve.

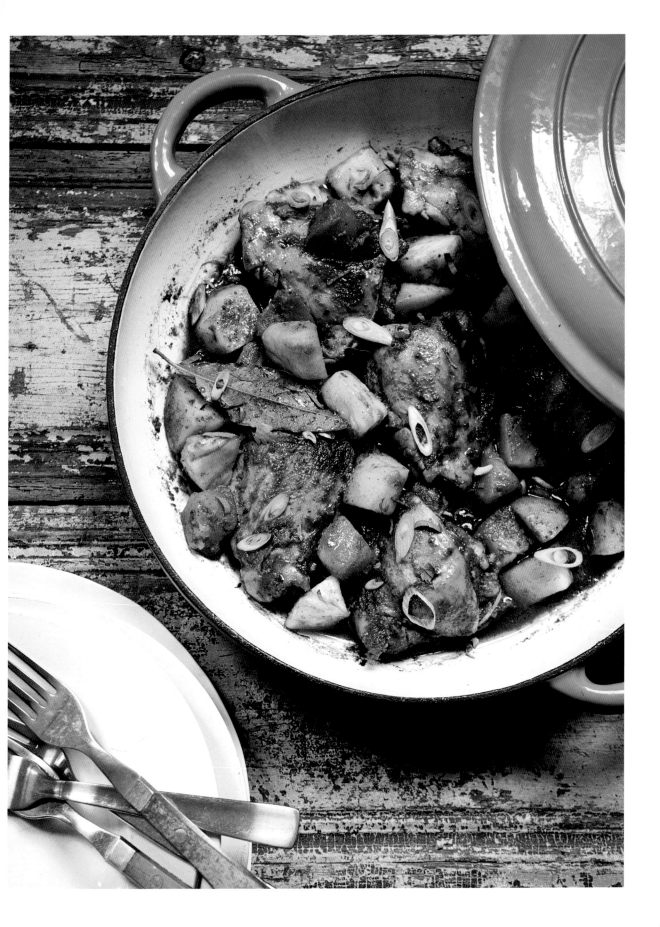

FUSION TANDOORI CHICKEN

214 calories per portion (2 drumsticks); 321 calories per portion (3 drumsticks)

We originally created this bit of fusion confusion for salmon but tried it with chicken and it was even better. You'll think that mixing tandoori spice, dill and capers sounds like a crazy idea but trust us, it really works! And it's so low cal you can serve some rice and salad alongside.

Serves 4–6
Prep: 10 minutes, plus at least 1 hour marinating time
Cooking time: 20–25 minutes

12 chicken drumsticks, skinned
100g low-fat natural yoghurt
2 tbsp chopped dill
2 tbsp capers
100g tandoori paste
1 tsp chilli powder (optional)
lemon wedges, to serve
flaked sea salt

Cut slashes in the flesh of the drumsticks, then put them in a bowl and season with salt. Put the yoghurt, dill and capers in a blender or food processor and blitz until the capers and dill are finely chopped. Mix this with the tandoori paste, and the chilli powder if you want some extra heat, then pour the lot over the chicken.

Make sure the paste covers the chicken – the best way to do this is to massage it into the cuts with your hands. Cover and leave to marinate for at least an hour, but preferably overnight.

When you're ready to cook the chicken, preheat the oven to its highest setting. Put a wire rack over a roasting tin. Take the drumsticks out of the marinade and place them on the rack. Bake for 20–25 minutes, turning occasionally, until the drumsticks are well cooked and starting to blacken in places.

Serve with lemon wedges to squeeze over the chicken.

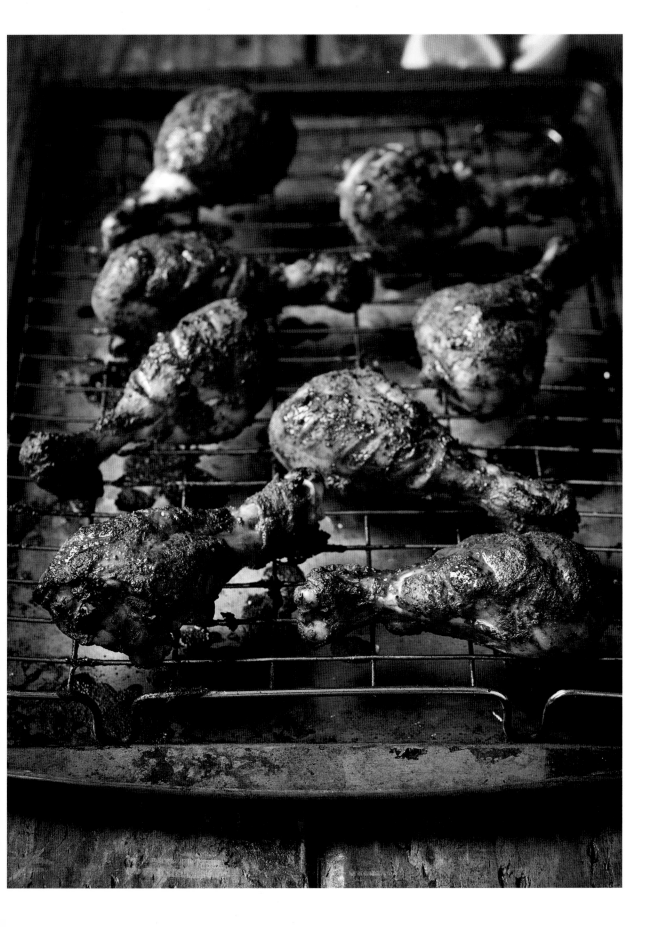

CHICKEN STIR-FRY

196 calories per portion

We learned so much when filming in Asia last year and we've tried to put our discoveries to good use in our latest healthy recipes. There are some traditional Chinese flavours in this stir-fry and as it's packed with veg you'll have generous servings. Once you've prepared everything for this dish it's cooked and on the table in the blink of an eye. Just be sure to cook the bean sprouts very briefly so they don't wilt and give off too much water in the wok.

Serves 4
Prep: 15 minutes, plus
20 minutes chilling
Cooking time: 6–8 minutes

2 chicken breasts, cut into
   thin strips
1 egg white
2 tsp cornflour
1 tbsp vegetable oil
300g tenderstem broccoli,
   halved lengthways
1 large red pepper, deseeded
   and cut into strips
100g mushrooms, wiped clean
   and cut in half
2 garlic cloves, finely sliced
15g chunk of fresh root ginger,
   peeled and finely chopped
2 red chillies, finely diced
   (deseeded if you like)
4 spring onions, sliced into rounds
225g can of water chestnuts,
   drained
150g bean sprouts
2 tbsp light soy sauce
2 tbsp rice wine (mirin)
4 tbsp chicken stock or water
1 tsp curry powder
½ tsp sesame oil
flaked sea salt
freshly ground black pepper

Put the chicken strips in a bowl. Whisk together the egg white and cornflour, making the paste as smooth as possible. Pour this over the chicken and mix thoroughly so the chicken is completely coated. Chill for 20 minutes in the fridge.

Heat the oil in a wok. Fry the chicken strips for one minute, until well browned and almost cooked through. Remove them from the wok, leaving behind as much oil as possible. Add the broccoli, red pepper and mushrooms and cook them over a high heat for 2 minutes, then add the garlic, ginger, chillies and sliced spring onions. Stir-fry for a further minute, then add the water chestnuts and bean sprouts.

Put the chicken back in the wok. Mix the soy sauce with the rice wine, chicken stock or water and curry powder in a bowl. Pour this mixture over the contents of the wok, season with salt and black pepper, then cook, stirring constantly for another 2 minutes.

Check that the chicken is cooked through, with no pinkness remaining, and cook for slightly longer if necessary. Just before serving, drizzle a little sesame oil on top.

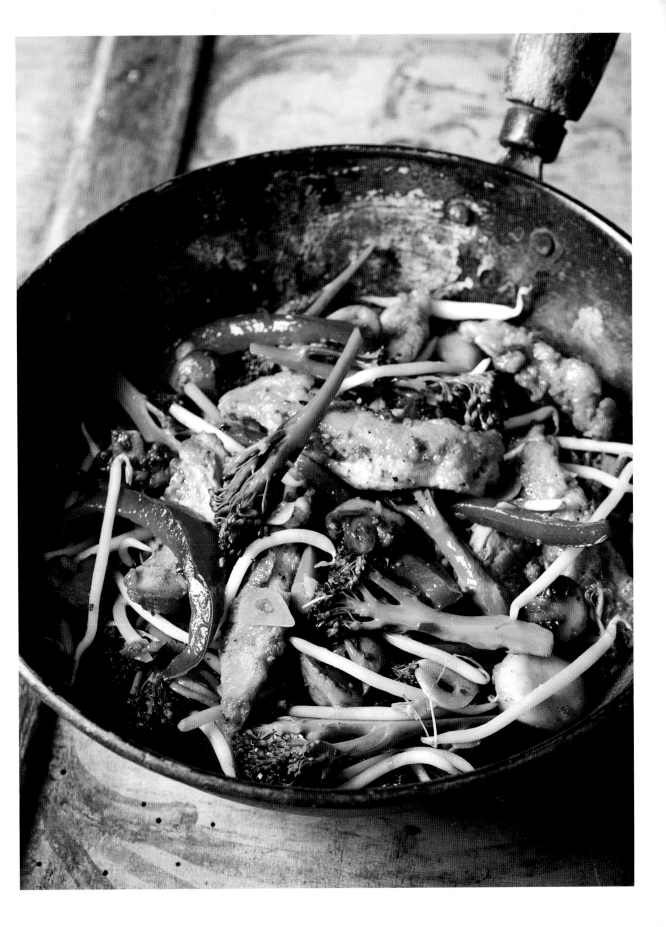

BEEF AND COCONUT CURRY

559 calories per portion (if serving 4); 447 calories (if serving 5)

This is based on an amazing dish we ate in a roadside café in Kerala back in 2005. We featured it in our curry book but this new version is lower in calories and just as good to eat. We've given details for a fab spice mix, which tastes brilliant, but if you're short of time and don't have all the spices, just use the garam masala with the fennel seeds and it will still be good. Great with roast cauli which adds just 25 calories per portion.

Serves 4–5
Prep: 20 minutes, plus at least 1 hour marinating
Cooking time: 2 hours 20 minutes

800g lean stewing steak, cut into chunks
2 onions, finely sliced
15g chunk of fresh root ginger, peeled and grated
4 garlic cloves, sliced
1 green chilli, deseeded and finely chopped
1 tbsp red wine vinegar
200ml coconut milk
1 tbsp vegetable oil
a handful of coriander leaves, chopped
sliced green chillies, to serve (optional)

Spice mix
4 cloves
2 tsp fennel seeds
1 tbsp coriander seeds
1 tsp chilli flakes
1 tsp ground turmeric
½ tsp ground cinnamon
2 tsp flaked sea salt
or
2 tsp fennel seeds
2 tsp garam masala
2 tsp flaked sea salt

First make the spice mix. Grind the cloves, fennel seeds, coriander seeds and chilli flakes in a spice grinder or pestle and mortar, then mix with the turmeric, cinnamon and salt. Alternatively, grind the fennel seeds and mix with the garam masala and salt. Put the beef in a large bowl and sprinkle over the spice mix. Add half the onions with the ginger, garlic, chilli and vinegar and mix well. Leave to marinate for at least an hour.

Put a heavy saucepan or heatproof casserole dish on top of the stove over a medium heat. Add the beef, along with its marinade, and pour in the coconut milk. Slowly bring to the boil, then turn the heat down, cover and cook on a very low heat for about an hour and a half, until the beef is tender. You will find that a lot of liquid comes out of the beef but don't worry – this is meant to happen.

When the beef is tender, remove the lid, turn up the heat to medium, then simmer the curry quite fiercely until all the liquid has evaporated. This will take up to half an hour and be sure to keep stirring every few minutes to make sure the meat doesn't catch on the bottom.

Once the liquid has reduced, heat the oil in a large frying pan. Add the remaining sliced onion and cook for a few minutes over a medium heat until the onion is golden brown. Add the beef mixture and continue to fry for 5–6 minutes until the meat is well browned and looks rich and gorgeous. Sprinkle with chopped coriander and chillies, if using, then serve with roasted spiced cauliflower.

Roast spiced cauliflower

Preheat the oven to 200°C/Fan 180°C/Gas 6. Bring a large pan of water to the boil and add the cauliflower florets. Cook for 2 minutes, then drain and leave to dry out in the colander.

Give the seeds a light pounding with a pestle and mortar or bash them with a rolling pin. Put the cauliflower in a roasting dish and toss with the vegetable oil. Sprinkle over the spices and the lime zest and juice, then season. Roast in the oven for about 15 minutes, until the cauliflower has started to brown round the edges. It should still be slightly firm.

Roast spiced cauliflower
½ head of cauliflower, broken into
    small florets
1 tsp vegetable oil
1 tsp nigella seeds (optional)
1 tsp cumin seeds
1 tsp coriander seeds
1 tsp mustard seeds (optional)
grated zest and juice of 1 lime
flaked sea salt
freshly ground black pepper

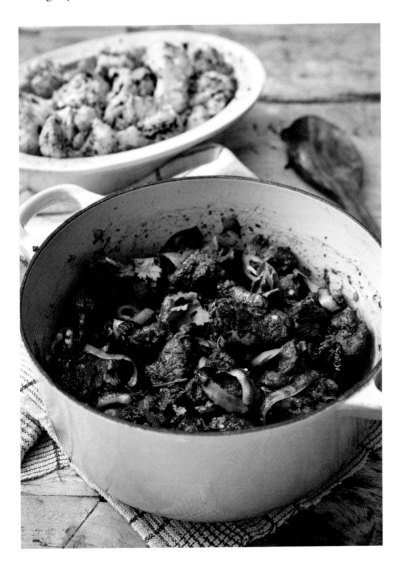

WEEKEND FEASTS

Weekends can be tricky when you're trying to lose a bit of weight. We know what it's like – you want to have a few friends over or to treat the family but you don't want to stray too far from your diet. With our weekend feasts you can keep everyone happy. We've included a few low-cal dishes you can enjoy as starters for a special dinner, such as piri piri prawns and our super scallop dish. Then you might like to serve up steak and kidney pie, coq au vin or our fab turkey crown roast, all carefully calorie counted. Delight your chums and keep yourself on track.

PIRI PIRI PRAWNS

130 calories per portion

These succulent prawns with a hit of chilli make a great starter for a special meal and can be cooked on a barbecue or indoors on a griddle pan. You'll need some bamboo or metal skewers. If you're a real chilli fiend you could add a couple of chopped bird's eye chillies to the marinade.

Serves 4
Prep: 15 minutes, plus marinating
Cooking time: 4–6 minutes

600g large peeled tiger prawns,
    deveined if necessary
lemon wedges, to serve

Marinade
4 plump red chillies, deseeded
    and roughly chopped
4 garlic cloves, peeled
20g bunch of flatleaf parsley
    (with stalks)
freshly squeezed juice of 2 lemons
    (about 65ml)
2 tbsp white wine vinegar
1 tsp smoked paprika
1 tsp oregano
1 tsp caster sugar
2 tsp flaked sea salt

To make the marinade, put all the ingredients in a food processor and blitz until everything is chopped quite finely and well combined.

Rinse the prawns in cold water and drain well, then put them in a bowl and cover with the marinade. Stir thoroughly to make sure the prawns are completely coated. Cover the bowl with cling film and leave the prawns to marinate in the fridge for at least a couple of hours. You can leave them overnight if you like.

If you're using bamboo skewers, soak them in water for half an hour before using to prevent them from burning. Thread the prawns on to the skewers. When your barbecue or griddle is hot enough, cook the prawns for 2–3 minutes on each side, until they have turned pink and opaque and have charred slightly. Be careful not to overcook them, though. Serve with lemon wedges – try popping them on the grill for a few minutes. They look great and produce lots of juice.

Top tip from us – these prawns are best eaten with your fingers!

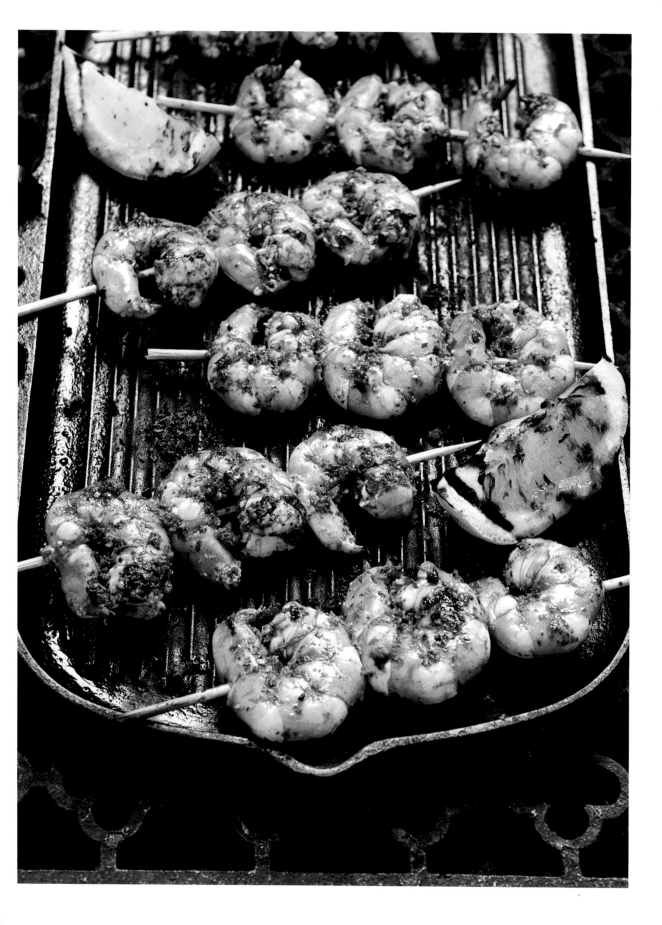

SCALLOPS WITH CORAL SAUCE
AND CAULIFLOWER PURÉE

142 calories per portion

We know that some people chuck away the coral from scallops. Seems a bit of a waste to us, as they're very tasty. Try our trick of whipping the corals up into a nice colourful topping for your scallops in this dish, which makes a cracking dinner party starter.

Serves 4 as a starter
Prep: 10 minutes
Cooking time: 15–20 minutes

12 scallops, with corals
1 tsp vegetable oil
1 shallot, finely chopped
4 tbsp fat-free natural yoghurt
pinch of cayenne
squeeze of lemon juice
oil, for spraying
pea shoots, for serving (optional)
flaked sea salt
freshly ground black pepper

Cauliflower purée
½ head of cauliflower, broken
   into florets
1 tbsp fat-free natural yoghurt
flaked sea salt

To make the cauliflower purée, bring a saucepan of water to the boil and add salt. Add the cauliflower and simmer for about 5 minutes, until it's soft. Strain and leave the cauliflower to drain for a few minutes. Blitz the cauli in a blender and add the yoghurt to make a purée. Tip this back into the pan and cover to keep it warm while you make the coral sauce and cook the scallops.

Separate the scallops from the corals and pull off the membrane. Heat the oil in a small frying pan and cook the shallot over a medium heat until it's soft and starting to caramelise. Turn the heat up towards the end of the cooking time to allow the shallot to brown more, but be careful not to let it burn.

Remove the shallot from the frying pan and add all the corals. Fry for a minute on each side, then remove them from the pan. Add a splash of water to the frying pan and stir, scraping up any brown bits of coral or shallot.

Put the shallot, corals, any liquid from the frying pan and the yoghurt into a blender. Season with salt and pepper and a pinch of cayenne, then blitz until smooth. Add a tiny squeeze of lemon juice and push the sauce through a sieve into a small saucepan to make it super-smooth. Heat gently while you sear the scallops.

Spritz a large frying pan with oil and put it over a medium heat. Add the scallops and sear for a couple of minutes on each side, pressing them down with a spatula so they take on a good colour.

Serve the scallops on small mounds of the cauliflower purée and top with spoonfuls of coral sauce. Sprinkle with pea shoots if you like.

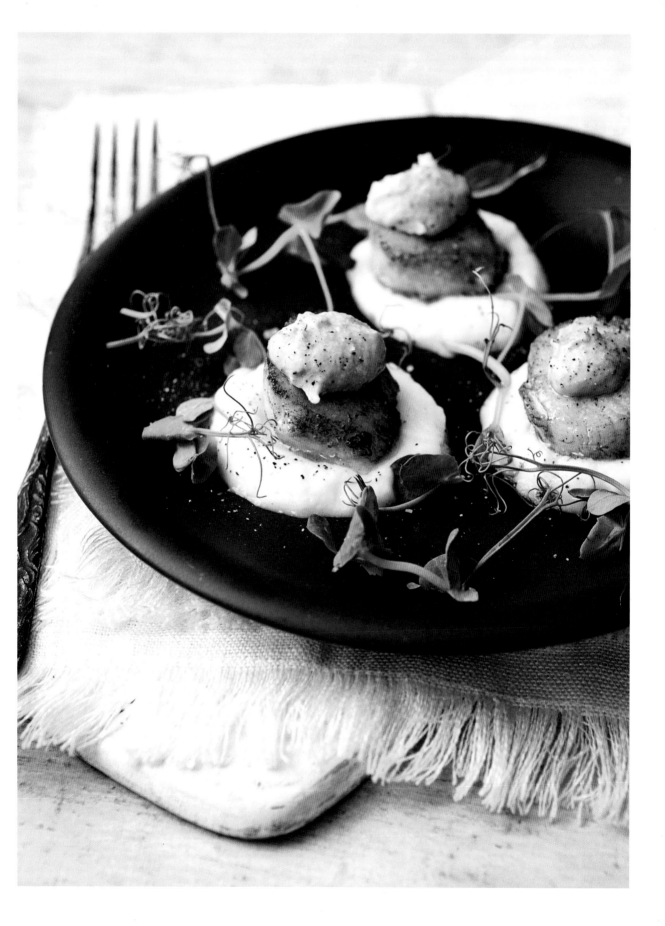

LETTUCE OR CHICORY CUPS WITH SMOKED DUCK AND ORANGE

37 calories per cup

Serve these little duck delights as a light starter or as canapés with drinks – we might be watching our weight but we're still dead posh. Use chicory or little gem lettuce leaves or some of each.

Makes 12
Prep: 10–15 minutes

1–2 heads of chicory or little gem
   lettuces
1 orange
175g smoked duck, skin removed
1 mild red chilli, finely diced
small bunch of fresh coriander,
   leaves only

Dressing
juice from segmenting the orange
1 tbsp olive oil
1 tsp sherry vinegar
1 tsp mustard
1 tsp honey
flaked sea salt
freshly ground black pepper

Cut the base off the chicory or little gems and separate out the best-shaped leaves. The leaves need to look fairly compact and cup-like, so they can hold the rest of the ingredients and should be of a size that can be eaten in one mouthful, so trim as necessary. You can use any leftover leaves in a salad.

Slice the top and bottom off the orange and place it on a chopping board, resting it on one of the flat ends. Using a sharp knife, cut off the peel and pith, working your way around the fruit. Next, cut between the membranes to release the segments. Do this over a bowl to catch any juice, then squeeze the remaining membrane and the discarded pieces of skin to extract as much juice as possible.

Dice the smoked duck and mix it with the red chilli.

For the dressing, add the reserved orange juice to the other ingredients and whisk everything together well.

To assemble, put a generous 2 teaspoons of the duck and chilli mixture on each leaf. Top with a piece of orange, drizzle over some of the dressing and finally sprinkle over some chopped coriander. Serve at once.

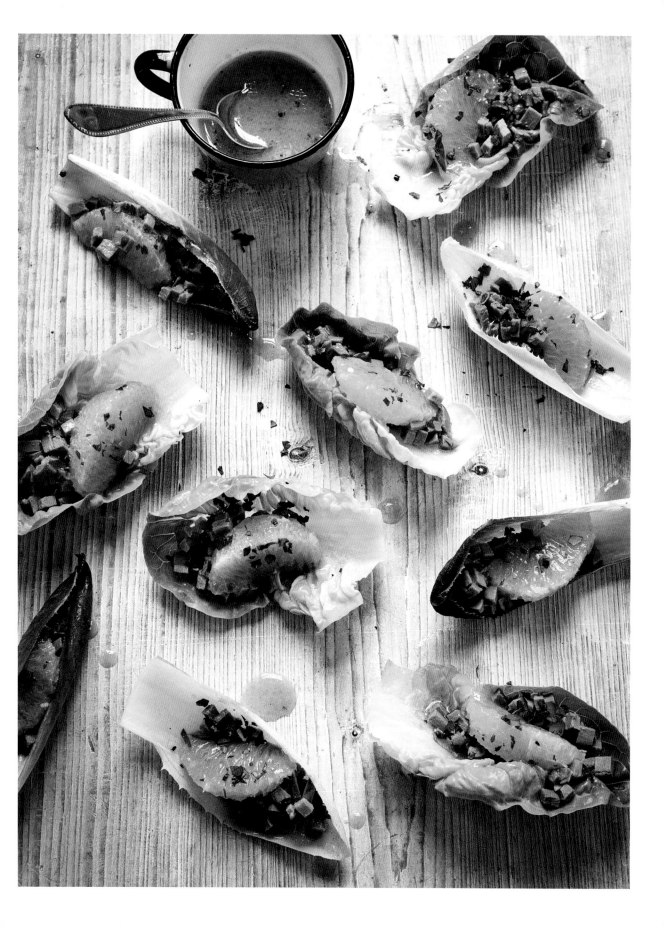

COQ AU VIN

400 calories per portion

This is our 'love in a transit' recipe rewritten to cut the calories but with no compromise on comfort or flavour. Lovely with some celeriac purée (see page 88) to soak up the juices.

Serves 4
Prep: 30 minutes, plus marinating
Cooking time: about 1 hour
30 minutes

300ml red wine
½ onion, finely chopped
1 carrot, peeled and finely diced
1 celery stick, trimmed and
     finely diced
4 garlic cloves, chopped
a few sprigs of thyme
2 bay leaves
1 clove
1 tbsp plain flour
4 bone-in, skinless chicken thighs
4 skinless chicken drumsticks
1 tbsp olive oil
4 rashers of back bacon, diced
400g button onions or shallots,
     peeled
250g button mushrooms,
     wiped clean
500ml chicken stock
1 tbsp redcurrant jelly
finely chopped parsley, to serve
flaked sea salt
freshly ground black pepper

Pour the wine into a saucepan and add the onion, carrot, celery, garlic, herbs and clove. Bring to the boil and boil fiercely for about 5 minutes to reduce the liquid a little and concentrate the flavours. Remove the pan from the heat and leave to cool. Put the chicken in a dish and once the liquid is cool, pour it over the chicken and leave to marinate for at least a few hours, or overnight if possible.

Spread the flour on a plate and season it with salt and pepper. Remove the chicken pieces from the red wine marinade and pat them dry with kitchen paper. Set the marinade aside for later. Dust the chicken pieces in flour and set aside.

Heat the oil in a large casserole dish. Add the bacon and brown it quickly, then transfer it to a plate with a slotted spoon and add the button onions, or shallots, and the mushrooms to the pan. Fry over a high heat for a minute, then turn the heat down and cook for about 10 minutes, stirring regularly, until the onions are nicely golden. Remove the onions and mushrooms from the dish, leaving behind as much oil as you can for browning the chicken. Add the chicken pieces and brown them on each side.

Put the bacon, onions and mushrooms back in the casserole dish, then strain the marinade through a sieve and pour this into the dish. Add the stock and redcurrant jelly. Bring everything to the boil, then turn the heat down to the lowest of simmers and cook, uncovered, for about an hour. After an hour everything should be tender and the sauce should be reduced.

If you want a slightly thicker sauce, remove the chicken, bacon and vegetables with a slotted spoon and put them on a warm serving dish. Bring the remaining liquid back to the boil and cook for a few minutes until it has reduced further, then pour it over the chicken. Check the seasoning and sprinkle with parsley before serving.

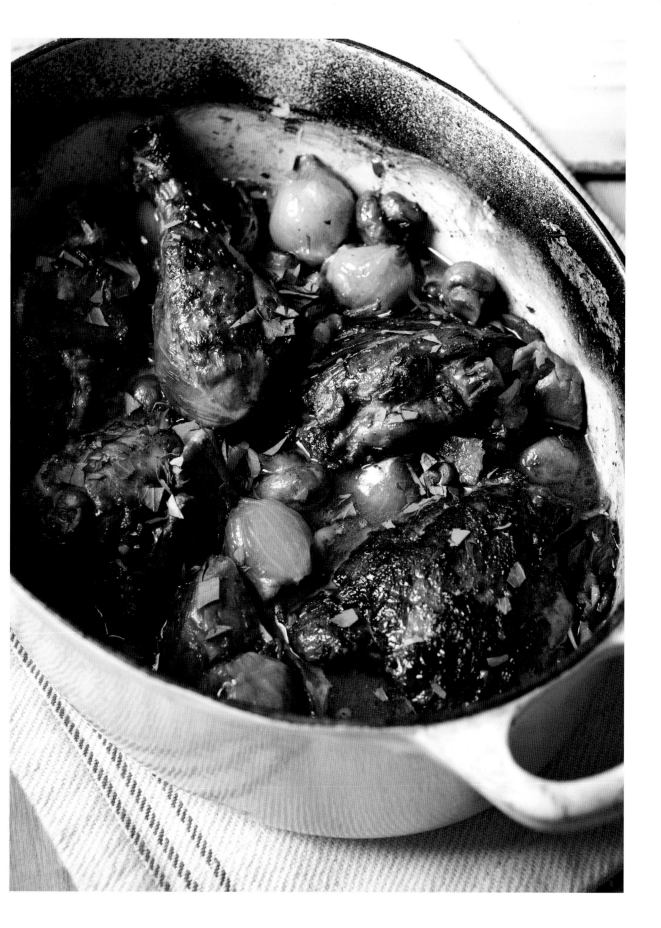

TUSCAN DEVIL'S CHICKEN

252 calories per portion (if serving 4); 168 per portion (if serving 6)

This is a great simple barbecue recipe or it can be cooked indoors if the weather is bad. It's also great cold for a picnic or lunch box.

Serves 4–6
Prep: 10 minutes, plus marinating
Cooking time: 10–15 minutes

12 boneless, skinless chicken thighs, trimmed of fat

Marinade
2 tbsp black peppercorns
juice of 2 lemons
1 tsp dried oregano
1 tsp olive oil

First, you need to flatten the chicken thighs. Open out a few so they are lying flat and place them between 2 large sheets of cling film. Now give them a good bashing with the smoother end of a meat mallet – or the bottom of a saucepan or a rolling pin will do fine. Repeat with the remaining thighs.

Put the chicken thighs in a bag with all the marinade ingredients. Close the top of the bag and massage the marinade well into the thighs, then leave them in the fridge for at least 2 hours or overnight if possible.

When you are ready to cook the chicken, heat your barbecue or a griddle pan on the hob. Brush most of the marinade off the chicken thighs and place them on the hot barbecue rack or griddle. Cook on one side for several minutes. When they are nicely charred on the underside, turn them over (you should be able to remove them quite easily at this point) and grill the other side until the chicken is completely cooked through and no trace of pinkness remains. As the thighs have been flattened, the cooking process shouldn't take longer than 10 minutes.

If you prefer, you can bake the chicken. Preheat the oven to 220°C/ Fan 200°C/Gas 7. Line a large baking tray with baking parchment and space the pieces of chicken out on the tray. Bake for about 15 minutes until the meat is cooked through, basting with any remaining marinade at intervals.

Great served with our tabbouleh (see page 124) or other salads.

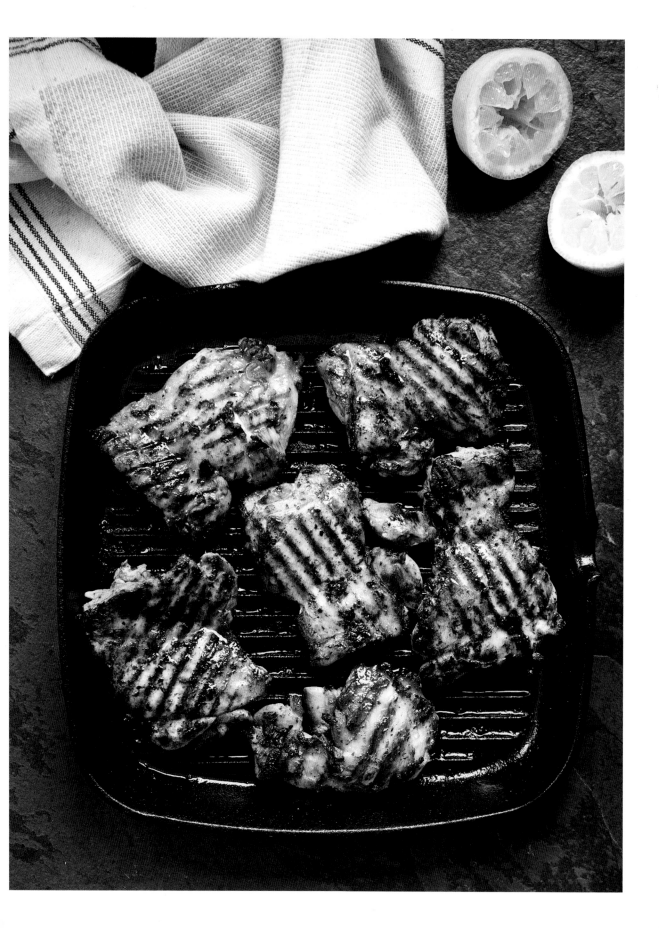

CHICKEN CHASSEUR

307 calories per portion

There's a reason why dishes like this are classics – it's because they're so good. Easy to make, this is a really tasty treat and delicious served with some celeriac purée to soak up the flavoursome juices.

Serves 4
Prep: 25 minutes
Cooking time: about 1 hour

8 bone-in, skinless chicken thighs,
   trimmed of fat
1 tbsp flour
2 tsp olive oil
2 shallots, finely chopped
2 garlic cloves, finely chopped
250g mushrooms, wiped clean
   and quartered
100ml white wine
1 tbsp tomato purée
300ml chicken stock
200g fresh tomatoes, peeled and
   chopped (or canned equivalent)
2 tbsp chopped tarragon leaves
flaked sea salt
freshly ground black pepper

Celeriac purée
1 large or 2 small celeriac, peeled
   and cut into small chunks (you
   need about 1kg peeled weight)
2 garlic cloves, roughly chopped
1 tbsp low-fat crème fraiche
flaked sea salt

FREEZE!

This can be frozen. Defrost thoroughly and reheat gently so you don't break up the chicken too much.

Before starting to cook, take each chicken thigh and place it bone-side up on your work surface. Cut either side of the bone so you can flatten the thigh out slightly – this helps it cook evenly. Season the chicken thighs with salt and pepper, then dust them with flour.

Heat a teaspoon of the oil in a large frying pan and add the chicken thighs. Cook them for a couple of minutes on each side until golden brown, then remove them from the pan and set aside – you might need to do this in a couple of batches. Turn the heat down and add the remaining teaspoon of olive oil to the pan. Add the shallots, garlic and mushrooms and fry over a very gentle heat for several minutes, stirring regularly, until everything has softened without taking on much colour.

Pour in the white wine and let it bubble, stirring with a wooden spoon to loosen any sticky bits from the bottom of the pan. Stir in the tomato purée, making sure it blends with the wine, then add the stock, tomatoes and tarragon. Put the chicken back in the pan. Simmer, uncovered, for about 40 minutes until the chicken is cooked through and tender, and the sauce has reduced. If it looks as though the pan is becoming too dry, add a splash of water. Serve with celeriac purée and some green veg or salad.

Celeriac purée

Put the celeriac and garlic in a medium-sized saucepan and cover with water. Season with a little salt. Bring up to simmering point, then cover and leave to cook over a low heat for about 15 minutes. Drain the celeriac and garlic in a colander, then tip everything back into the pan and mash well or purée with a stick blender. Stir in the crème fraiche, check the seasoning and serve.

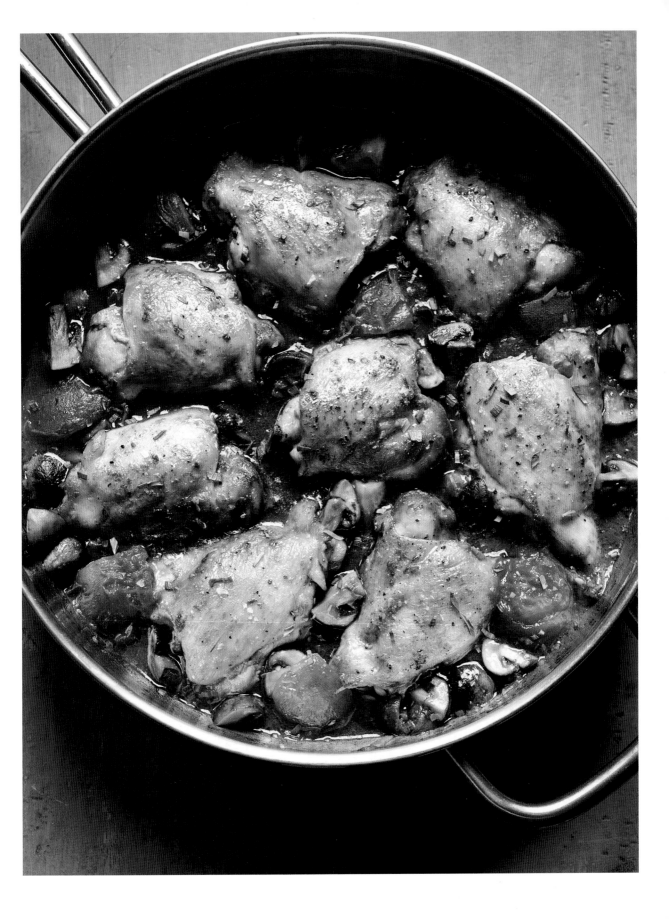

POT-ROAST PORK WITH CIDER AND APPLES

277 calories per portion

Lean pork meat is not high in calories, but don't kid yourself that crackling or pork fat can ever be low cal. It has to be trimmed off. Pork and apple work as well together as Fred and Ginger – or Si and Dave – and the cider in this recipe makes for a beautifully fragrant, yet light gravy. We find that it's best to use eating apples, such as Coxes, for this. Bramleys fall apart too much. The sauce is great as it is, but you can thicken it with a little arrowroot if you prefer.

Serves 6
Prep: 15 minutes
Cooking time: 1 hour
and 15–30 minutes

1 tbsp olive oil
1kg piece of rolled pork shoulder
    or loin, trimmed of fat
2 onions, sliced
6 garlic cloves, unpeeled
1 tsp dried sage or 1 tbsp fresh sage,
    chopped
2 bay leaves
300ml cider
2 eating apples, peeled,
    cored and sliced
flaked sea salt
freshly ground black pepper

Preheat the oven to 200°C/Fan 180°C/Gas 6.

Heat the oil in a large casserole dish. Season the pork with salt and black pepper, place it in the dish and brown it on all sides. Remove the pork and set it aside, turn down the heat and add the onions. Cook them slowly for about 10 minutes until they have softened but don't let them brown. If they start to catch, add a splash of water.

Put the pork back in the casserole dish and add the garlic and herbs. Pour in the cider. Cover the dish with a lid and place it in the preheated oven for 45 minutes. Remove the dish from the oven and add the apples, then put it back for another 15–30 minutes until the pork is cooked through and tender.

Transfer the pork to a warm serving dish and leave it to rest. Strain the cooking liquid, reserving the apples and onions. Remove the garlic, squish the flesh from the skins, then whisk it into the cooking liquid – chuck the skins away. You will have a very thin, creamy-looking gravy.

Serve the pork cut into thick slices, garnished with the onions and apples and a good glug of gravy.

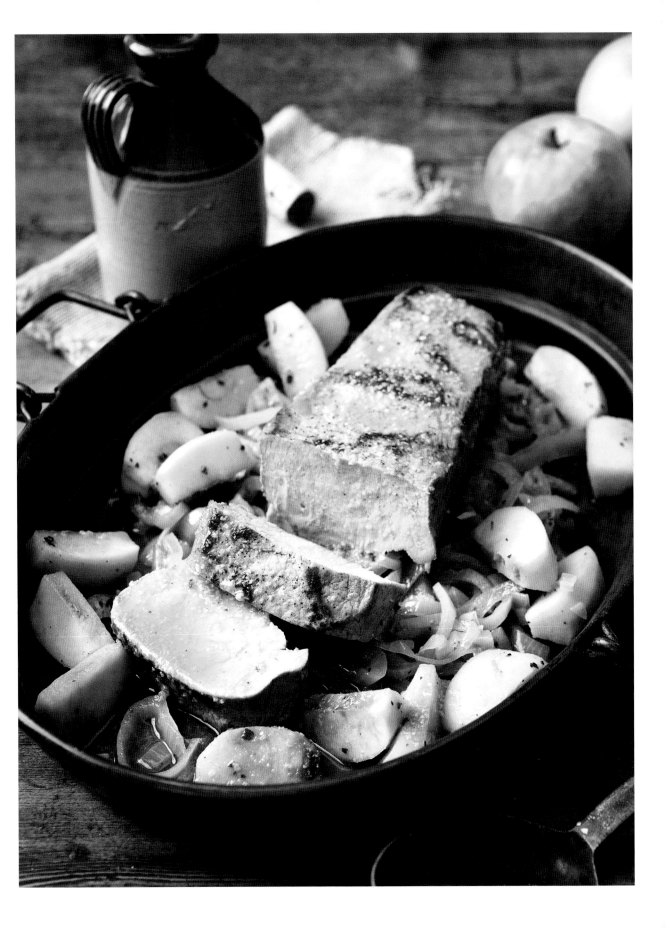

ROAST TURKEY CROWN WITH SWEET POTATO, MUSHROOM AND CHESTNUT STUFFING AND GRAVY

321 calories per portion (100g of turkey and all the trimmings);
373 calories per portion (150g of turkey and all the trimmings)

This is the answer to everyone who has been asking what to do for Christmas dinner or a big celebration when you're trying to watch the calories. Just don't gobble down too much!

Serves 6 (with leftovers)
Prep: 45 minutes
Cooking time: 1 hour 45 minutes

1 turkey crown (2–3kg, depending
   on how many you want to feed)
1 large onion, sliced widthways
   into even slices
1 large sprig of tarragon
150ml white wine
1 tsp flour (optional)
flaked sea salt
freshly ground black pepper

Stuffing
½ onion, finely chopped
2 celery sticks, finely chopped
100g mushrooms, wiped clean
   and finely chopped
150g sweet potato, finely chopped
100g chestnuts, finely chopped
   (vacuum-packed are fine)
2 rashers of streaky bacon, finely
   chopped
1 tsp chopped thyme leaves
1 tsp dried oregano

Roast potatoes and parsnips
600g potatoes
300g parsnips
oil, for spraying

First make the stuffing, chopping the vegetables and chestnuts in a food processor if you like. Heat a non-stick frying pan and add the bacon. Cook until some of the fat renders out, then add all the other ingredients, including the herbs and seasoning. Cook over a fairly low heat for about 10 minutes, until everything starts to soften, then turn up the heat and cook for a few more minutes to caramelise the veg a little. Remove the pan from the heat and leave the stuffing to cool. Weigh the stuffing and add this to the weight of the turkey so you can work out the cooking time.

Preheat the oven to its highest setting. Take the turkey out of the fridge half an hour before you want to cook it. Loosen the skin around the neck end (between the fattest part of the breasts). When the stuffing is cool, fill the neck cavity – it should hold all the stuffing. Pull the skin over tightly and secure it with a skewer. Put the onion slices in the middle of a roasting tin and add the tarragon. Lie the turkey crown on top, then pour in the wine and 150ml of water and season with salt and pepper.

Put the turkey in the oven and roast at the high temperature for 30 minutes. Turn the oven down to 180°C/Fan 160°C/Gas 4 and cook for another 12–15 minutes per kilogram. Make sure the turkey is cooked by piercing the thickest part with a skewer. The juices should run clear and the tip of the skewer should be almost too hot to touch. If the juices are still pink, cook for a little longer.

Remove the turkey and onions from the roasting tin, cover with foil and leave to rest for 20 minutes. The meat juices in the tin will be lovely as they are, so you can just put the tin over a low heat, stir well to lift any dark, caramelised bits, then strain into a warm jug.

If you want to thicken the gravy, pour off the juices, put the tin over a low heat and sprinkle over a teaspoon of flour. Stir, making sure you scrape up any of the bits sticking to the tin, then pour the liquid back in, a little at a time, until you have a thick gravy. Carve the turkey and serve with the gravy, stuffing, roast potatoes and parsnips and some green veg.

Roast potatoes and parsnips

Bring a saucepan of water to the boil. Add the potatoes and parsnips and simmer for 5 minutes to parboil. Drain the veg in a colander, then shake them around a bit to roughen up the edges. Tip them into a roasting tin or baking tray, then spritz with oil and season.

Put the potatoes and parsnips into the oven once the turkey has had its first 30 minutes at the high temperature. When you take the turkey out of the oven, whack the temperature up to 200°C/Fan 180°C/Gas 6 so the veg can finish cooking while the turkey rests.

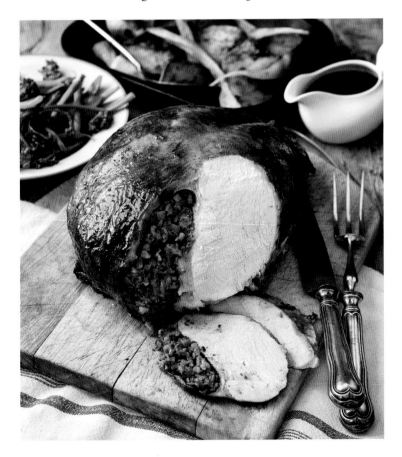

STEAK PIZZAIOLA

317 calories per portion (without cheese);
369 calories per portion (with cheese)

This is so easy to prepare and a real treat to eat. There are lots of different recipes for this dish, some including peppers, mushrooms and so on, but we prefer to keep it simple and enjoy the wonderful flavour combination of tomato sauce and steak. And if you like you can top it all off with a little melted cheese.

Serves 2
Prep: 15 minutes
Cooking time: 25–35 minutes

4 large very ripe tomatoes
1 tbsp olive oil
2 shallots, finely chopped
2 garlic cloves, crushed
1 tbsp fresh oregano or 1 tsp dried
    oregano
pinch of caster sugar (optional)
1 lean rump steak (about 325g),
    2cm thick
salad leaves, to serve
25g hard cheese such as Cheddar
    or Gruyère, very thinly sliced
    (optional)
flaked sea salt
freshly ground black pepper

First peel the tomatoes. To do this, score a small cross in the base of each and put them in a small bowl. Cover the tomatoes with freshly boiled hot water, count to 10, then remove them from the water. The skins will slip off easily. Chop the tomatoes and set them aside.

Heat the olive oil in a non-stick frying pan. Add the shallots and fry over a medium heat for several minutes until they're soft and translucent. Add the garlic and cook for 2 minutes more, stirring regularly. Now add the oregano and tomatoes and bring everything to the boil. Simmer the sauce for about 15 minutes until well reduced, then taste for seasoning and add a little sugar if needed.

Trim as much fat off the steak as you can, then season the meat with salt and pepper. Cut the steak in half. Heat a griddle pan for several minutes until it is as hot as you can get it, then add the steaks. Grill them for 2–3 minutes on each side or according to taste. Transfer them to a board and leave to rest for a few minutes.

Once the steaks have rested, strain any meat juices into the tomato sauce. Cook the sauce for another minute to allow the juices to combine. Lay the steaks on warm plates, then spoon over the sauce and serve immediately, garnished with some salad leaves.

If you want to add cheese, heat the grill to its highest setting while you're cooking the steaks, but cook the steaks for a minute less on the second side. When the steaks have rested, put them in an ovenproof dish, cover with tomato sauce, then top with the cheese. Put the dish under the hot grill until the cheese has melted and started to brown.

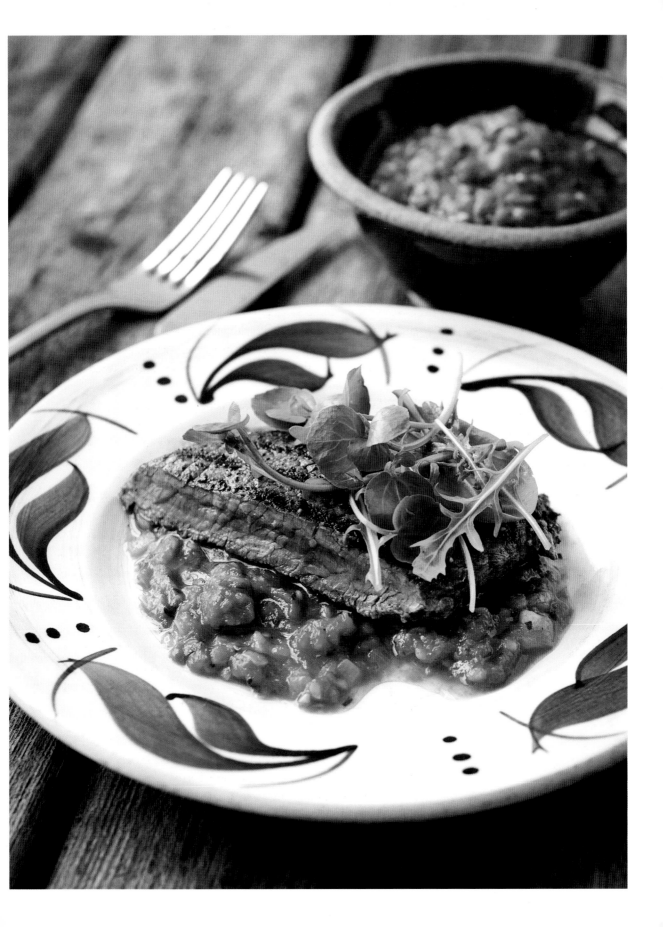

STEAK AND KIDNEY PIE

400 calories per portion

This is one of our favourite pies, made with our special potato pastry – the next instalment in our quest for a great but low-cal pie crust. If you're not keen on kidneys, you can use mushrooms instead, which will cut the calorie count down a little. You'll need about 200g of button mushrooms. Cut them in half and add them towards the end of the onions' cooking time.

Serves 6
Prep: 40 minutes, plus pastry chilling time
Cooking time: 2 hours 30 minutes

Filling
750g braising steak, trimmed of
    all fat and cut into 2.5cm cubes
3 lambs' kidneys, cores removed
    and meat diced
1 tbsp flour
1 tsp mustard powder (optional)
1 tbsp vegetable oil
2 large onions, sliced lengthways
100ml red wine
a few sprigs of thyme
1 bay leaf
500ml beef stock
1 tsp Worcestershire sauce
flaked sea salt
freshly ground black pepper

Pastry
275g floury potatoes, preferably
    Maris Pipers or King Edwards
40g chilled butter, diced
80g plain flour
1–2 tbsp semi-skimmed milk
1 egg, lightly beaten, to glaze
pinch of salt

First make the mash for the pastry. Peel the potatoes and cut them into chunks of about 3cm. Put them in a large saucepan, cover with cold water and bring to the boil. Cook for 10–15 minutes or until very tender. Drain the potatoes in a colander, tip them back into the saucepan, then mash until smooth – don't add any butter or milk. Leave to cool.

To make the filling, put the cubes of beef and kidneys in a bowl. Mix the flour with the mustard powder, if using, and season with salt and pepper. Sprinkle this on to the meat and turn the meat over lightly with your hands, making sure that it all gets a covering.

Heat the oil in a large casserole dish. Add the onions and cook over a very low heat until they're quite soft and translucent. Remove them from the dish. Turn the heat up and add the meat, stirring very quickly until it's coloured all over. Leave the heat turned up and pour in the red wine. Allow it to bubble up, then stir, making sure you scrape up any brown bits stuck to the base of the pan. Add the thyme sprigs and bay leaf, then pour in the beef stock. Add the Worcestershire sauce and tip the onions back into the pan.

Bring everything to the boil, then cover and turn the heat down as low as you can. Simmer gently for about an hour and a half until the meat is tender. Remove the meat and onions from the casserole dish with a slotted spoon and transfer to an oval pie dish. Turn the heat up and boil the remaining liquid until it is thick and gravy-like, then pour this over the meat and onions. Put a pie funnel in the centre of the pie dish if you have one.

To make the pastry, rub the butter into the flour in a bowl, then add 200g of mash and 1 tablespoon of the milk. Season with a pinch of salt. Work everything together into a dough, handling it as lightly as possible. If it's too dry, add a touch more milk, but only a teaspoon at a time. When you have a smooth dough, roll it into a ball, cover it with cling film and chill for at least half an hour.

Preheat the oven to 200°C/Fan 180°C/Gas 6. Roll the pastry out on a lightly floured work surface, until it is large enough to cover your pie dish. It will be fairly thin, about 3mm, but it will be robust enough that it won't break when you lift it. Wet the rim of the pie dish with water. Carefully lift the pastry using the rolling pin and place it over the pie, pressing the edges firmly around the rim of the dish. Cut a hole for the pie funnel if you're using one. For a good colour, glaze the pie with beaten egg. Bake the pie in the preheated oven for 40–45 minutes until the top is a deep golden brown.

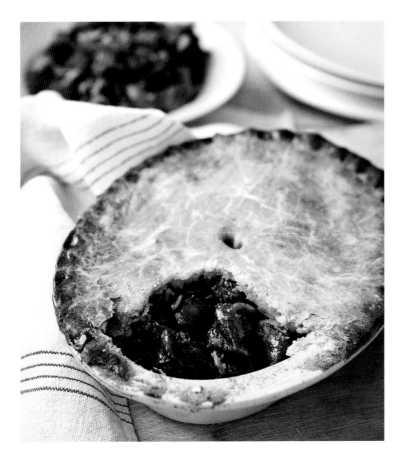

CHILLI STEAK SALAD

322 calories per portion (if serving 2); 161 calories per portion (if serving 4)

Like lots of other people, we loved the Thai beef salad in our last book so we've come up with a variation on the theme. Cutting the steak into strips makes it look like you're getting more, which is always encouraging.

**Serves 2 as main course
or 4 as a starter**
Prep: 15 minutes
Cooking time: 4–6 minutes

1 sirloin steak, about 400g
100g salad leaves, such as rocket,
    watercress, baby spinach
12 radishes, quartered
½ cucumber, halved and cut into
    very thin rounds
4 spring onions, halved widthways
    then shredded
small bunch of coriander, chopped
flaked sea salt
freshly ground black pepper

Dressing
2 garlic cloves, finely chopped
15g chunk of fresh root ginger,
    peeled and grated
1–2 red chillies, finely chopped
    (deseeded if you like)
2 tbsp fish sauce
freshly squeezed juice of 1 lime
1 tsp caster sugar

First make the dressing. Mix together all the ingredients, stirring until the sugar has dissolved. Taste and season with salt and pepper, then set aside.

Heat a griddle pan until it is as hot as you can get it. Trim the steak of any visible fat and season with salt and pepper. Cook the steak on the griddle for 2–3 minutes on each side or according to taste – although medium rare is probably best for this dish.

Put the steak on a board and leave it to rest for a few minutes. Arrange the salad ingredients on a large platter, or on individual plates if you prefer.

Slice the steak into thin strips, then pour any meat juices into the dressing and stir. Arrange the meat on top of the salad, then pour over the salad dressing. Serve at once.

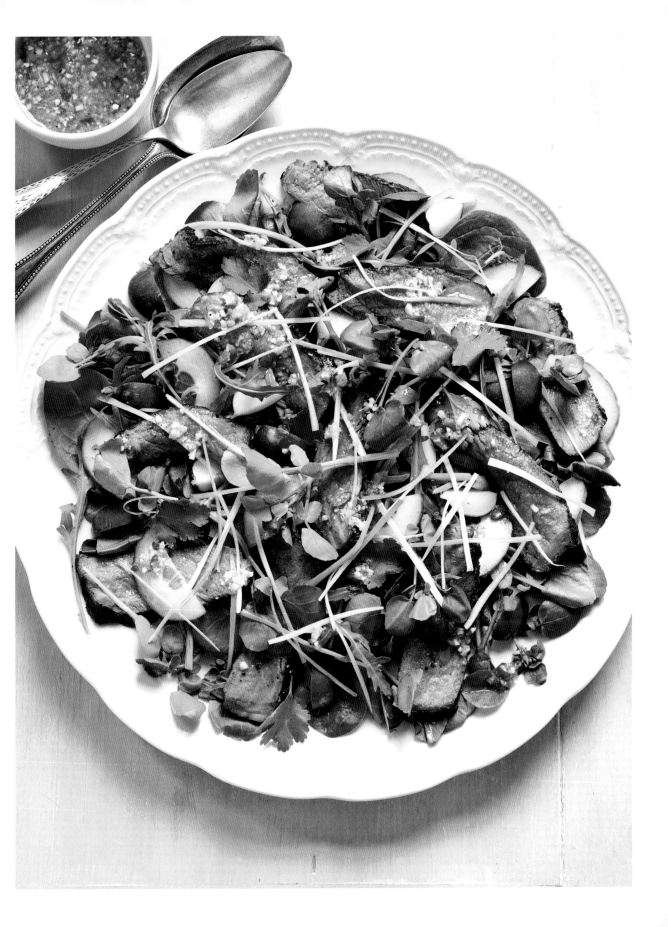

COMFORT CLASSICS

There are some great old favourites in this chapter –
dishes such as warming tomato soup and Scotch broth
that are always good to come home too. They're like a
lovely cuddle for your tummy. We reckon pasta is the
most comforting, heart-warming food of all so we've
included some of our latest spaghetti suggestions.
And then there are pies. We can't live without our pies
and we now have an amazing new pastry recipe that
you just have to try. It contains mashed potato instead
of some of the flour, which incredibly makes
it lower in calories – surprising and delicious!

TOMATO SOUP

171 calories per portion

*Our tomato soup is really rich, creamy and flavoursome – but there's no cream in it,
no sugar, just lots of veg. It's a great way of getting the kids to have some of their
five a day too. The fennel seeds add an extra tang of flavour but if you don't have any,
or don't like them, just leave them out. You could also chill this soup and keep it
in the fridge to enjoy as a snack, like gazpacho.*

Serves 4
Prep: 15 minutes
Cooking time: 25–35 minutes

1 tbsp olive oil
1 onion, diced
1 celery stick, trimmed and diced
1 large carrot, peeled and diced
1 leek, trimmed and thinly sliced
100g butternut squash, peeled
  and diced
200g celeriac, peeled and diced
1 tsp fennel seeds, ground
  (optional)
2 garlic cloves, finely chopped
50g red lentils
1.2 litres vegetable or chicken stock
400g can of tomatoes
handful of basil leaves, shredded
flaked sea salt
freshly ground black pepper

Heat the olive oil in a large saucepan and add the onion, celery, carrot, leek, squash and celeriac. Sauté over a fairly high heat, stirring regularly, until the vegetables are starting to brown slightly around the edges and give off a sweet aroma.

Add the fennel seeds, if using, and the garlic and sauté for another 2 minutes. Add the red lentils and pour over the stock, then season with salt and pepper. Simmer for 10 minutes.

Add the tomatoes and simmer for another 10–15 minutes until the lentils are completely soft. Add the basil and let it wilt into the soup, then remove the pan from the heat. Purée the soup until smooth, adding more stock or water if it seems too thick for your liking. Taste for seasoning before serving and adjust if necessary.

FREEZE!

Ideal for freezing in individual portions, ready to defrost for a super-quick lunch.

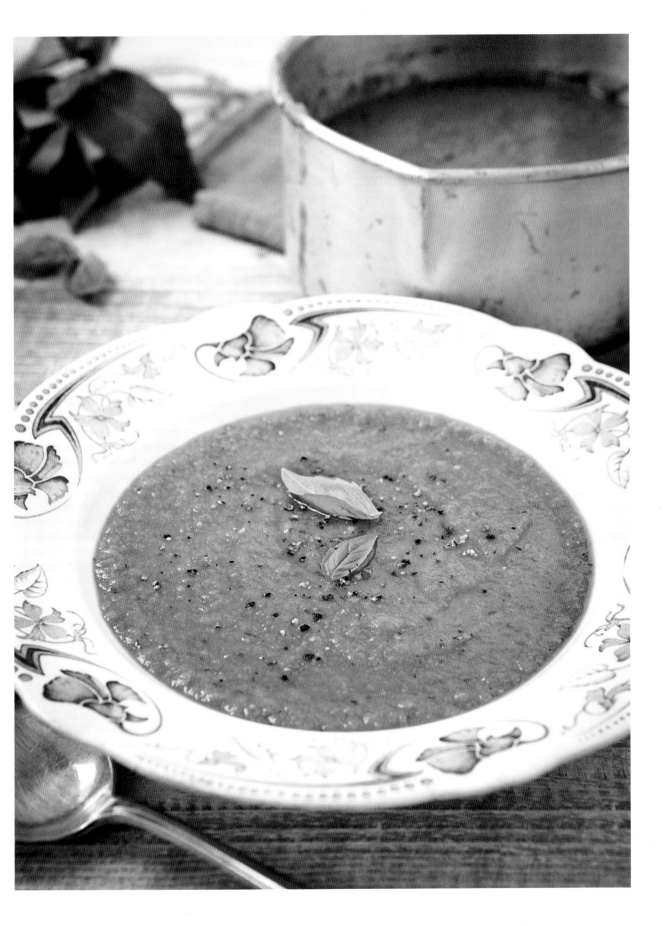

SCOTCH BROTH

240 calories per portion (if serving 6); 180 calories per portion (if serving 8)

As you diet, you begin to see your ribs again and this hearty soup will stick to them. Some recipes for this gutsy, nourishing Scottish classic use just lamb stock while others include neck fillet or other cuts. Neck is fatty so we use diced lamb leg meat to add flavour and texture to the soup, along with loads of luscious veg and barley. We think it's best to soak the peas overnight, then boil them for ten minutes before adding them to the soup to be on the safe side. You don't want to end up with tough little green bullets in your soup!

Serves 6–8
Prep: 20 minutes, plus soaking time
Cooking time: 1 hour 30 minutes

50g split green peas, soaked
    overnight
400g lean lamb leg meat,
    finely diced
1.2 litres lamb stock or water
50g pearl barley
4 carrots, peeled and finely diced
2 onions, finely diced
2 celery sticks, trimmed and
    finely diced
½ swede, peeled and finely diced
1 large turnip, peeled and finely
    diced
1 sprig of thyme
1 bay leaf
½ cabbage, shredded (white, green
    or savoy)
2 leeks, halved lengthways and
    finely sliced
flaked sea salt
freshly ground black pepper

Soak the split green peas overnight in plenty of water. When you are ready to start making the Scotch broth, drain the peas and put them in a saucepan. Cover with cold water, bring to the boil and boil hard for 10 minutes, then drain and set aside. The peas are now ready to use.

Put the lamb in a large saucepan or casserole dish, cover it with the stock and bring everything to the boil. Skim off any brown foam that collects on the surface and keep doing this until the foam turns white. Add the pearl barley, boiled split peas, carrots, onions, celery, swede, turnips and herbs, then season with salt and pepper and bring back to the boil. Turn the heat down to a low simmer and cook gently for an hour, adding more liquid if necessary.

Add the cabbage and leeks and simmer for another 15 minutes until they are just tender. Serve the Scotch broth in deep bowls.

FREEZE!

Despite containing a lot of vegetables with a high water content, this can be frozen, as the veg are diced very small. Their texture will be slightly affected when defrosted, but it's not as noticeable as it would be if they were cut into large chunks.

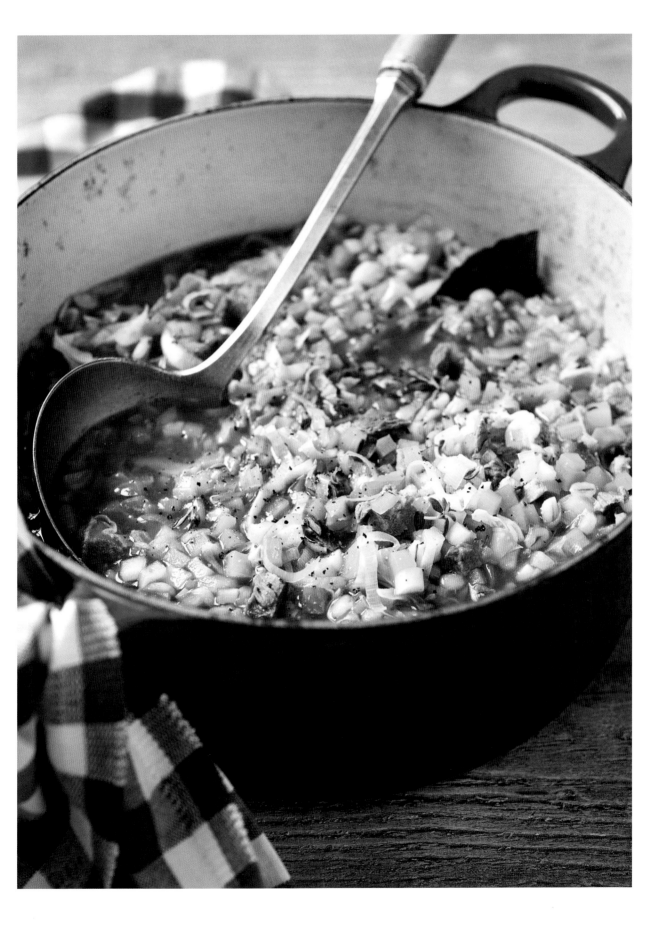

BROAD BEAN PILAF

218 calories per portion (if serving 4); 145 calories per portion (if serving 6)
Chicken version: 310 calories per portion (if serving 4); 207 calories (if serving 6)

Dill goes beautifully with broad beans in this lovely comforting rice recipe, which is inspired by a dish we cooked during a very early Hairy Biker trip to Turkey. It's easy to make, but we have to say that unless you have really tiny young beans, it's worth going the extra mile and removing the greyish-green skin that covers each bean. It does make them taste better.

Serves 4 as a main; 6 as a side dish
Prep: 20 minutes, plus marinating time for chicken
Cooking time: about 25 minutes

1 tsp vegetable oil
1 small onion, finely diced
1 small courgette (or half a big one), cut into small dice
1 small piece of cinnamon stick
5 cardamom pods, lightly crushed
1 tsp cumin
½ tsp black pepper
175g basmati rice, well rinsed
300ml vegetable or chicken stock
250g broad beans (fresh or frozen)
a large bunch of parsley, chopped
a small bunch of dill, chopped
flaked sea salt
freshly ground black pepper

Chicken pilaf
ingredients as above, plus
75ml low-fat natural yoghurt
freshly squeezed juice of ½ lemon
a pinch of cinnamon
15g chunk of fresh root ginger, finely grated
4 boneless, skinless chicken thighs, cut into bite-sized pieces

Heat the oil in a saucepan. Add the onion, courgette and spices, then cook over a medium heat for a few minutes until you can smell the wonderful aroma of the spices.

Add the rice and give everything a good stir to make sure the rice is well coated. Pour in the stock and season well with salt. Bring to the boil, then turn down the heat to a gentle simmer, cover the pan and leave for 10 minutes. While the rice is cooking, remove the skins from the beans – this is known as double podding! Using your thumbnail, slit the skin and pop out the bright green bean. Set the beans aside. If you're using frozen beans, defrost them first.

When the rice has been cooking for 10 minutes, add the broad beans. Leave to cook for another 5 minutes, then turn off the heat and leave to stand for 5 minutes. Fluff up the rice with a fork, turning it over gently so the broad beans mix well with everything else. Stir in the herbs, season with salt and pepper if needed and pile the pilaf on to a large serving plate.

Chicken pilaf
Mix together the yoghurt, lemon juice, cinnamon and ginger in a bowl. Season the chicken with salt and pepper, then add the pieces to the marinade in the bowl and leave for an hour.

Follow the recipe as above, but add the chicken, scraped of most of the marinade, just before the rice and stir it for a couple of minutes so it mixes well with the other ingredients and starts to brown slightly. Then add the rice and proceed as before.

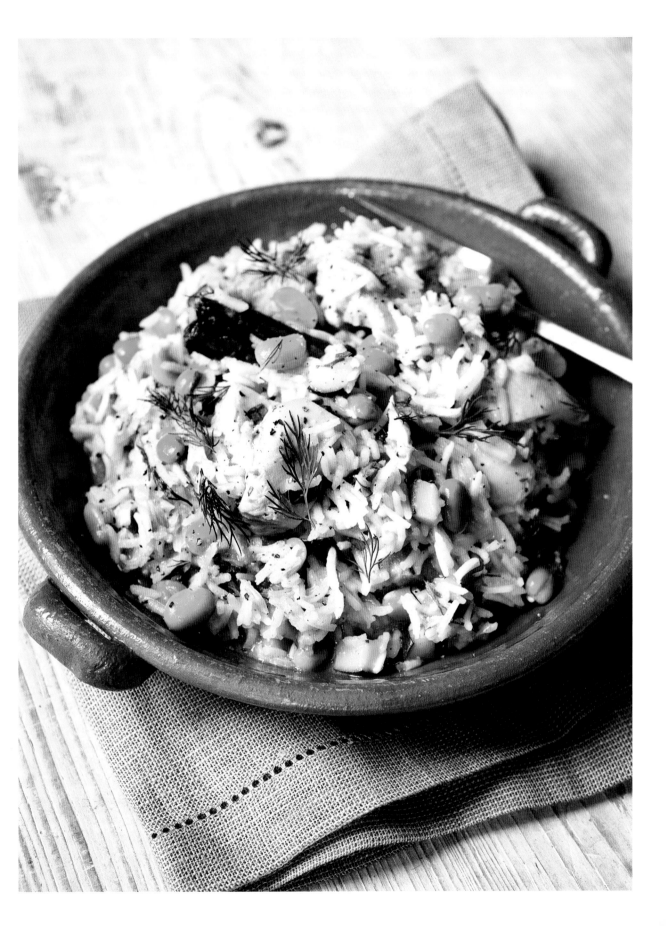

CREAMY CHICKEN AND TARRAGON POTS WITH ROSEMARY POTATO WEDGES

chicken: 231 calories per portion; potato wedges: 109 calories per portion

We love that loads of our readers are sending us their own great recipes to try so we decided to hold a competition and print the winner. Here's what Amy Hulyer says about her recipe: 'a tasty, tempting pot of creamy deliciousness with all the yum factor of a Great British chicken pie, but none of the calories of puff pastry or double cream'. Congratulations Amy, we totally agree. You'll need some deep ramekins for the chicken pots.

Serves: 3
Prep time: 20 minutes
Cooking time: 40–45 minutes

1 tsp olive oil
2 medium leeks, trimmed and
    sliced into 5mm rings
2 garlic cloves, crushed
3 rashers of lean smoked bacon
2 boneless, skinless chicken breasts
200ml chicken stock
small bunch of fresh tarragon or
    1 tsp dried tarragon
2 tbsp low-fat crème fraiche
30g reduced-fat mature Cheddar
    cheese, grated
freshly ground black pepper

Rosemary-roasted new potato wedges
400g new potatoes
    (about 6 large ones), cut into
    quarters lengthways
1 tsp vegetable oil
a large sprig of rosemary
1 garlic clove, crushed
flaked sea salt
freshly ground black pepper

Place a large non-stick frying pan over a medium heat. Add the olive oil and leek slices and cook for 3 minutes until the leek is starting to soften. Add the crushed garlic and cook for another 2 minutes.

Preheat the oven to 200°C/Fan 180°C/Gas 6. Trim any fat off the bacon and chicken and dice the meat. Add it all to the pan with the leeks, stir and cook over a moderate heat for 5–10 minutes until the chicken is no longer pink. Add the stock to the pan and reduce the heat a little. Cook for 10 minutes until nearly all the stock has reduced and the leeks are completely soft. Turn the heat right down and add the tarragon and crème fraiche, then cook for another 2 minutes. Season with a good grind of pepper.

Spoon the mixture into ramekins and top with the grated cheese. Place the pots on a baking tray and cook in the oven for 15 minutes, until bubbling and golden. Allow to cool for a couple of minutes before serving with green veg and roasted new potato wedges.

Rosemary-roasted new potato wedges
Preheat the oven to 200°C/Fan 180°C/Gas 6 and put a large non-stick baking tray in the oven to heat up. Bring a pan of water to the boil, add the potato wedges and cook for 4 minutes. Drain and put the wedges in a bowl with the oil and rosemary, then season generously. Mix everything together until the potatoes are well coated, then transfer to the heated baking tray in a single layer. Cook for 20 minutes, then add the garlic, give them a good shake around and cook for another 10–15 minutes until golden and crispy.

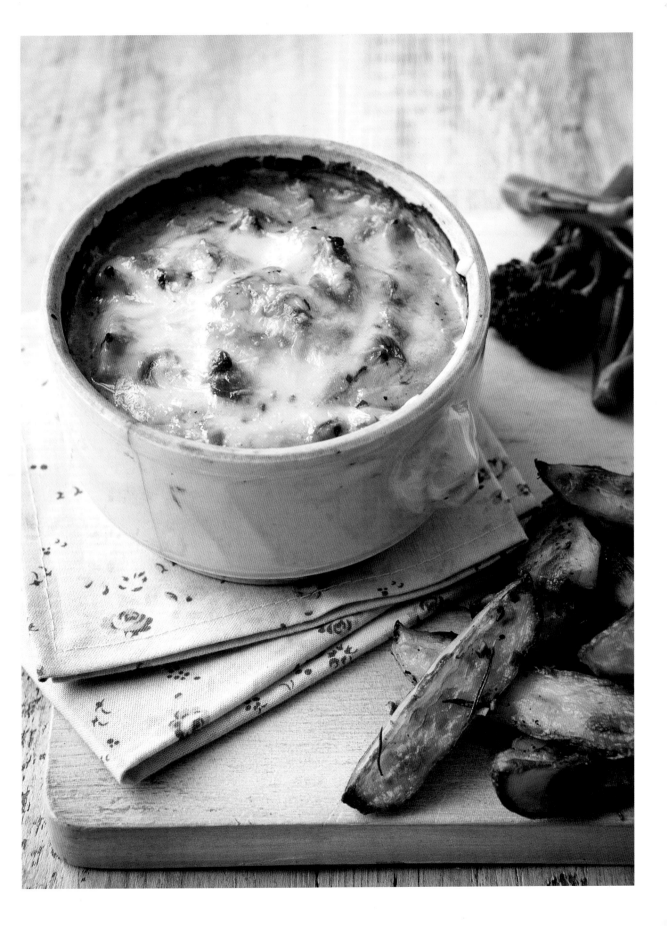

PASTA WITH CLAMS AND BACON

295 calories per portion

Proper Italian this is, but it's made with tinned clams that you can get in any supermarket. Shellfish and bacon go brilliantly together and using bacon means you don't need much oil. It adds loads of flavour too.

Serves: 4
Prep time: 10 minutes
Cooking time: 10–12 minutes

200g spaghetti
1 tbsp olive oil
2 slices of lean bacon, finely chopped
1 shallot or small onion, finely chopped
3 garlic cloves, finely chopped
1 tsp chilli flakes (or according to taste)
100ml white wine
280g can of clams in brine, drained
2 tbsp chopped flatleaf parsley
flaked sea salt
freshly ground black pepper

Bring a large saucepan of water to the boil. Add the spaghetti, stir well and bring the water back to the boil. Cook the pasta for 10–12 minutes until tender, or according to the packet instructions, stirring occasionally.

While the spaghetti is cooking, heat the oil in a large frying pan over a medium heat. Add the bacon and fry it until crisp and brown. Remove the bacon from the pan and set it aside. Turn the heat down, add the chopped shallot or onion and cook slowly until soft and translucent. Add the garlic and chilli flakes and cook for another 2 minutes, then pour in the wine and simmer for a couple of minutes.

Drain the clams, reserving some of their liquor. Add 50ml of this liquor, along with the clams, to the frying pan, then put the bacon back in the pan. Taste for seasoning and add salt if necessary and a grinding of black pepper.

Drain the pasta in a colander, then tip it into the frying pan. Turn it over so it is all completely covered with the sauce, then serve sprinkled with plenty of parsley.

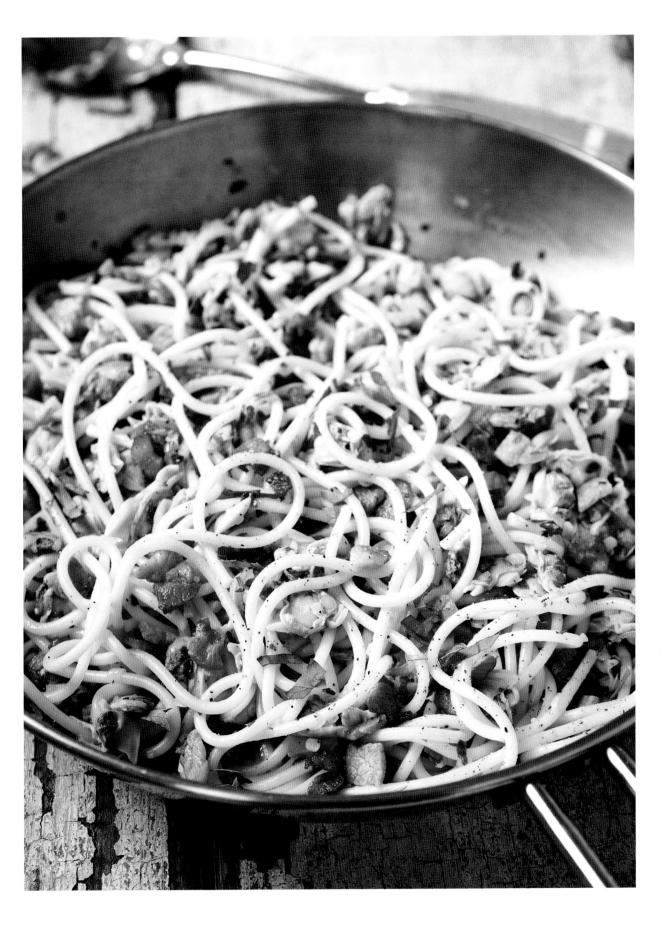

PASTA WITH SUMMER VEGETABLES AND PARMA HAM

305 calories per portion

This is a deliciously light summery pasta and a welcome change from rich tomato-based sauces. You could use finely sliced runner beans instead of broad beans if you like, and if you leave out the Parma ham this makes an excellent vegetarian dish.

Serves 4
Prep: 20 minutes
Cooking time: 25–30 minutes

75g broad beans (fresh or frozen)
1 tbsp olive oil
1 leek, trimmed and finely sliced
1 garlic clove
2 little gem lettuces, trimmed and cut lengthways
100g asparagus spears, cut into 4cm lengths
100g peas (fresh or frozen)
1 tbsp fresh tarragon, chopped
50ml white wine
150ml vegetable stock or water
2 tbsp low-fat crème fraiche
200g short pasta, such as farfalle
4 slices of Parma ham
a few leaves of basil, torn
25g Parmesan cheese, grated
flaked sea salt
freshly ground black pepper

Bring a saucepan of water to the boil, add the broad beans and boil them for 1 minute. Remove the pan from the heat, drain the beans and plunge them into a bowl of ice water for a couple of minutes, then drain again. To remove the tough skins from the beans, slit the skin of each one with your thumbnail and pop out the bright green bean. Set the beans aside.

Heat the olive oil in a large saucepan. Add the slices of leek and cook for a few minutes until they're starting to soften. Add the garlic, cook for another minute, then add all the remaining vegetables, and the tarragon, spreading them evenly over the base of the saucepan. Season with salt and black pepper.

Pour in the white wine, let it simmer for a couple of minutes, then add the stock or water. Put the lid on the pan and simmer the veg for about 10 minutes, until the little gems have wilted down. Stir in the crème fraiche and simmer for another couple of minutes.

Meanwhile, bring a large saucepan of water to the boil. Add the pasta, stir well and bring the water back to the boil. Cook the pasta for 10–12 minutes until tender, or according to the packet instructions, stirring occasionally. Drain.

Stir the pasta into the pan with the sauce. Tear the slices of Parma ham into shreds and stir those in, too, with the basil. Sprinkle with the grated Parmesan and serve.

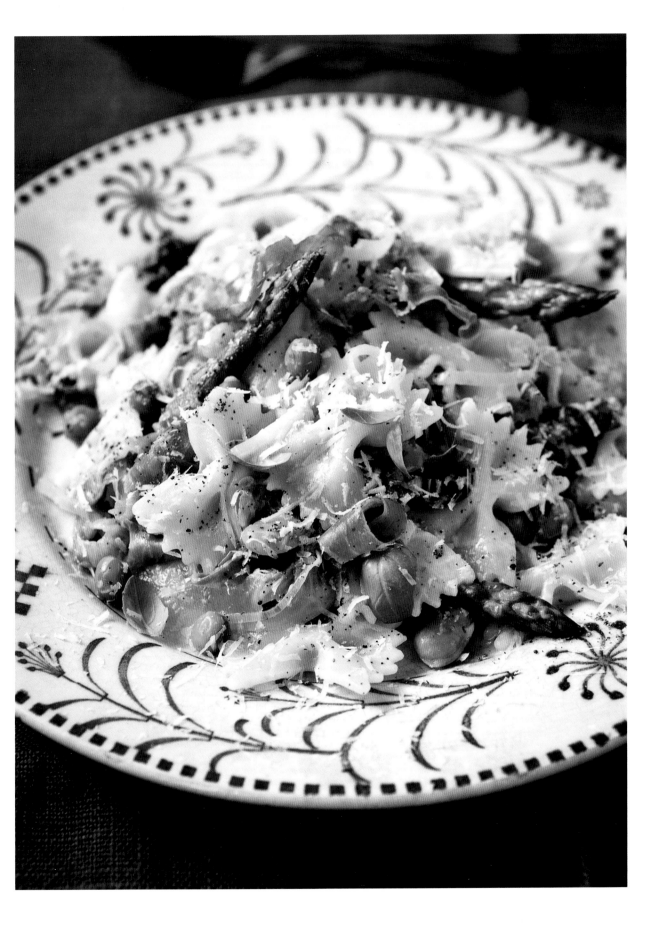

SPAGHETTI WITH PRAWNS AND COURGETTES

250 calories per portion

By popular demand we've included plenty of pasta in this book and this recipe makes us glad we did. It's a super-quick dish that you can put together in not much longer than it takes the spaghetti to cook. There's plenty of great flavours so no need for Parmesan – only adds calories. This doesn't have any sauce as such, and the whole thing is loosened with a ladleful of the cooking liquid. The pasta gives out just enough starch to thicken the water slightly.

Serves 4
Prep: 10 minutes
Cooking time: up to 15 minutes

200g spaghetti
1 tbsp olive oil
1 onion, finely chopped
1 large or 2 medium-sized
    courgettes, diced
2 garlic cloves, finely chopped
freshly grated zest of 1 lemon
2 tbsp capers
200g brown shrimp or cooked,
    peeled North Atlantic prawns,
    defrosted
a fine grating of nutmeg
handful of basil leaves, roughly torn
flaked sea salt
freshly ground black pepper

Bring a large saucepan of water to the boil and add a pinch of salt. Add the spaghetti, stir well and bring the water back to the boil. Cook the pasta for 10–12 minutes until tender, or according to the packet instructions, stirring occasionally.

While the pasta is cooking, heat the olive oil in a large frying pan. Add the onion and courgettes and cook until the onion is soft and the courgettes have started to soften around the edges – you don't want them to break down any more than that. Add the garlic and cook for another couple of minutes, then add the lemon zest and capers and season with lots of black pepper.

When the pasta is done, drain it in a colander, reserving a jugful of the cooking liquid. Add the shrimp or prawns to the frying pan, then a small ladleful of the pasta cooking liquid. Grate over a little nutmeg. Allow the sauce to bubble for a few moments, then add the pasta and the basil. Turn everything over so it is all thoroughly combined. If the dish seems too dry, add a little more cooking liquid. Serve immediately.

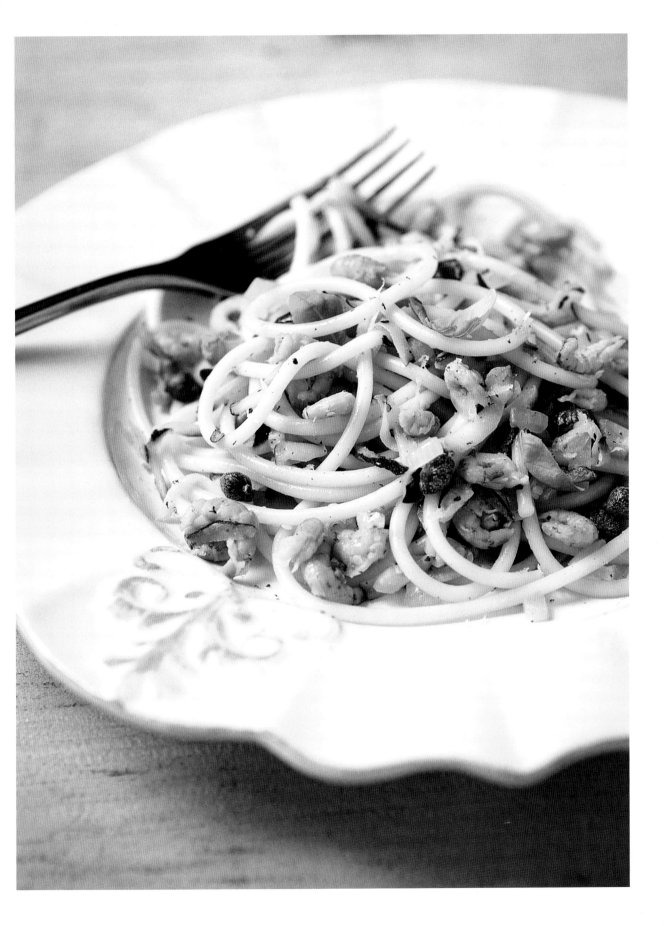

IRISH STEW

500 calories per portion

A traditional Irish stew is made with lamb on the bone or neck fillet, but neck is very fatty, so is high in calories. We prefer double chops – Barnsley chops – or leg steaks, which are fairly lean, and using meat on the bone gives extra flavour. The marrow helps the texture of the dish too. One thing you can do to reduce the fat – and calorie count – if you have time, is to cook the dish the night before up to the point of adding the potatoes, then chill. The next day, skim off the fat, which will have solidified, then reheat and add the potatoes as below.

Serves 4 generously
Prep: 20 minutes
Cooking time: 1 hour
20–30 minutes

4 Barnsley chops or leg steaks
1 tbsp oil
2 large onions, sliced
4 large carrots, peeled and sliced
    widthways on the diagonal
2 bay leaves
a sprig of thyme
a sprig of parsley
750ml–1 litre lamb or chicken
    stock, to cover
600g potatoes, peeled and
    thickly sliced
2 tbsp chopped parsley, to serve
    (optional)
flaked sea salt
freshly ground black pepper

Trim the meat of any excess fat. If using chops, you can also pull off the skin if you like, as there will be some fat just under it.

Heat the oil in a large casserole dish. Add the lamb and brown it well on both sides. Remove the lamb from the dish and add the onions and carrots. Cook, while stirring, for a couple of minutes, then add the herbs and put the lamb back in the dish. Pour in the stock, making sure the lamb and vegetables are just covered, and season with salt and pepper.

Cover the casserole dish and bring the stew to the boil, then turn the heat down and simmer for about 45 minutes. By this time the lamb should be well on its way to being tender. Add the potato slices in a layer on the top and simmer until they are tender and starting to break down – this should take about 20 minutes. Sprinkle with parsley before serving if you like.

FREEZE!

If you want to freeze this stew, prepare it up to and including the stage of simmering for 45 minutes, then cool and freeze. When you want to use it, defrost and reheat gently, then add the potatoes and finish cooking as above.

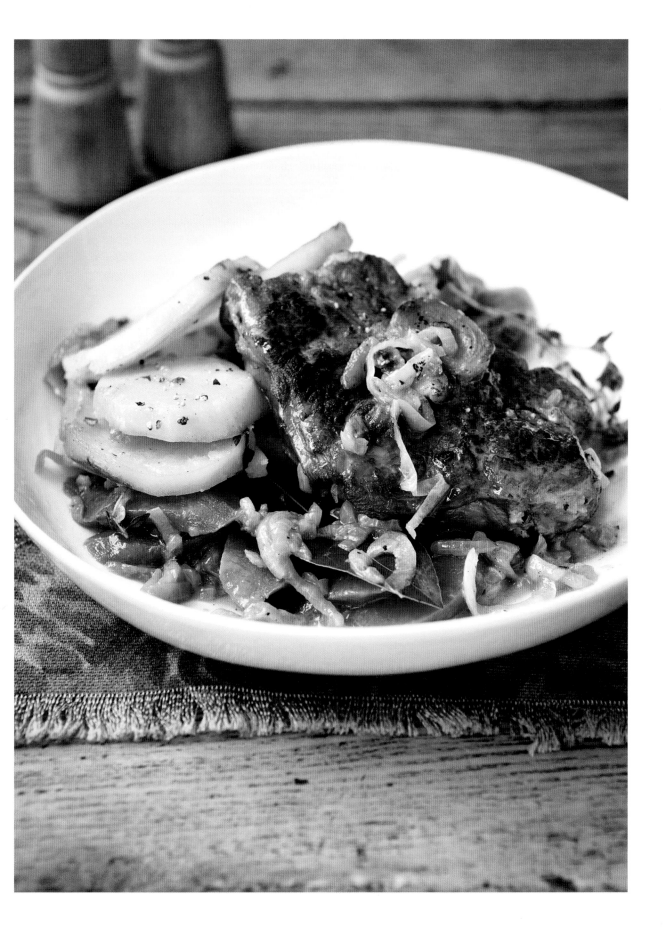

MINCED BEEF PLATE PIE

439 calories per portion (if serving 4); 351 calories per portion (if serving 5); 293 calories per portion (if serving 6)

One thing we're really pleased about is that we've managed to lose weight while still enjoying our favourite foods – such as pies. Surprisingly, potatoes contain fewer calories than flour so by using some mash in this pastry you can also include butter, which gives it great taste and texture. We call this a 'cut and come again pie', but beware of making too many visits if you want to stay sylphlike.

Serves 4–6
Prep: 30 minutes, plus chilling time for pastry
Cooking time: about 1 hour 15 minutes

Filling
250g lean beef mince
2 onions, sliced
2 carrots, peeled and cut into small dice
100g swede, peeled weight, cut into small dice
2 celery sticks, trimmed and diced
400g can of brown lentils, drained
1 tsp dried oregano
1 tsp finely chopped thyme
1 tbsp anchovy paste (optional)
1 tbsp tomato purée
300ml beef stock
flaked sea salt
freshly ground black pepper

Pastry
275g floury potatoes, preferably Maris Pipers or King Edwards
40g chilled butter, diced
80g plain flour
1–2 tbsp semi-skimmed milk
1 egg, lightly beaten, to glaze
pinch of salt

Make the pastry as for our steak and kidney pie on pages 96–97. Wrap it in cling film and leave it to chill for at least half an hour.

Meanwhile, make the filling, put the mince, onions, carrots, swede and celery in a large frying pan. Dry-fry, stirring constantly until the beef has browned and make sure you break up any clumps of meat. Add the lentils, herbs, anchovy paste (if using), tomato purée and stock. Stir to mix everything well, then bring to the boil and season with salt and pepper. Cover the pan and simmer for about 20 minutes or until the vegetables have softened. Set aside to cool.

Preheat the oven to 200°C/Fan 180°C/Gas 6. Tip the filling into a round pie plate or dish. Roll the pastry out on a lightly floured work surface until it is large enough to cover your pie plate. It will be fairly thin, about 3mm, but should be robust enough not to break when you lift it.

Wet the rim of the pie plate with water. Carefully lift the pastry using the rolling pin and place it over the pie, pressing the edges firmly around the rim. For a good colour, glaze the pie with some lightly beaten egg.

Bake in the preheated oven for 40–45 minutes until the pastry is cooked and a lovely golden colour. Serve with some freshly cooked green vegetables.

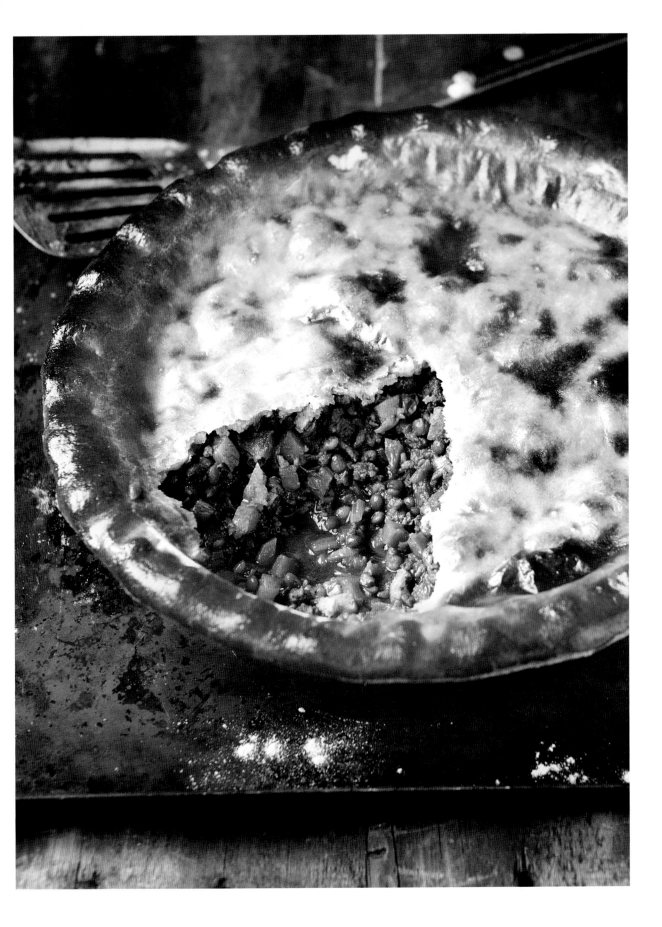

VEGGIE WONDERS

We love our vegetables and we've learned that they can be the stars of the show – not just something to add a bit of colour on the plate. Recipes like our aubergine bake and Greek roast vegetables can be a meal in themselves, as well as going beautifully with some grilled meat or chicken. We've also come up with some deliciously hearty salads, such as our versions of Middle Eastern tabbouleh and fattoush, that will really tickle your taste buds.

AUBERGINE BAKE

205 calories per portion (with one ball of mozzarella); 269 calories with two balls

Our low-cal version of an Italian classic – melanzane parmigiana – makes a comforting veggie supper dish. Aubergines are low in calories, despite their chunky, meaty feel, but the dish usually contains lots of oil. We've cut right back on the oil but there's still plenty of tasty sauce. Use one or two balls of mozzarella as you like, but remember that more mozz means more calories.

Serves 4
Prep: 15–20 minutes
Cooking time: 1 hour 15 minutes
(if cooking aubergines in 1 batch)

4 large aubergines,
    sliced into 1cm rounds
oil, for spraying
a handful of basil leaves,
    roughly torn
1 or 2 balls of half-fat mozzarella

Tomato sauce
1 tbsp olive oil
1 onion, finely chopped
2 cloves garlic, finely chopped
1 tsp oregano
small pinch of cinnamon
small pinch of sugar
200ml red wine
2 x 400g cans of chopped tomatoes
flaked sea salt
freshly ground black pepper

Preheat the oven to 200°C/Fan 180°C/Gas 6. You may need to cook the aubergines in a couple of batches. Line 2 large baking trays with non-stick baking parchment. Arrange the slices of aubergine on the trays, then mist them very lightly with oil – you will probably need about 3 sprays per tray.

Put the trays in the oven and roast the aubergine slices until they are soft and the flesh is golden brown in patches. This will take about 40–45 minutes. Remove the aubergines from the oven and set them aside to cool while you cook the rest of the slices in the same way.

Meanwhile make the tomato sauce. Heat the olive oil in a large saucepan. Add the onion and fry over a low heat until soft and translucent. Add the garlic and cook for another 2 minutes. Sprinkle over the oregano, cinnamon and sugar and give everything a quick stir. Pour in the red wine and turn up the heat, then simmer quite briskly until the liquid has reduced by about half. Add the tomatoes and season with salt and pepper, then simmer for at least 20 minutes, until the sauce has reduced and thickened.

Take a large ovenproof baking dish and spread a little of the tomato sauce on the bottom. Cover with a layer of aubergines and some roughly torn basil, then continue adding layers of sauce and aubergines until you have used everything up – you should have at least 3 layers of aubergines. Finish with a thin layer of tomato sauce. Slice the mozzarella as thinly as you can and arrange it over the aubergines and sauce. It doesn't matter if there are gaps, it will spread a little during cooking. Put the dish in the oven and bake for 30 minutes until the aubergines are very tender and the mozzarella has melted and browned a little. Serve with a green salad.

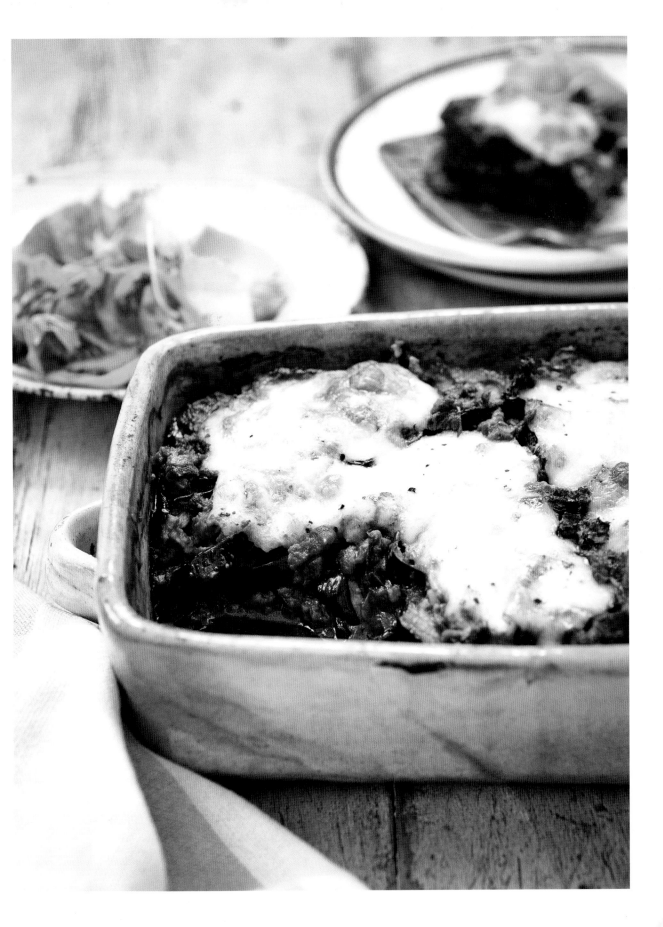

TABBOULEH

101 calories per portion (if serving 4); 68 calories per portion (if serving 6)

An authentic tabbouleh contains very little bulgur wheat but lots and lots of herbs, and ours is no exception. This is great on its own, with a group of other salad dishes or with some grilled chicken. The celeriac adds extra texture, but if you don't like it – or can't get hold of any – just use an extra courgette.

Serves 4–6
Prep: 15 minutes, plus
20 minutes soaking time

1 red onion, finely chopped
30g bulgur wheat
100g celeriac, peeled
2 courgettes
200g large, ripe red tomatoes,
    finely chopped
1 red pepper, deseeded and
    finely diced
a large bunch of flatleaf parsley,
    finely sliced (not chopped)
a small bunch of mint, leaves only,
    finely sliced
flaked sea salt

Dressing
1 tbsp olive oil
juice of 1 lemon
pinch of cinnamon
1 tsp ground cumin
flaked sea salt
freshly ground black pepper

Put the finely chopped red onion in a bowl, sprinkle with some salt and cover with cold water. Leave to stand for 20 minutes. This takes the harshness out of the onions and makes the flavour more mellow. Soak the bulgur wheat in a bowl of just-boiled water for 5 minutes, then drain and set aside.

Cut the celeriac into chunks. Top and tail the courgettes and cut them into chunks too. Put the celeriac in a food processor and pulse a few times, then add the courgettes and pulse again until everything is the size of large breadcrumbs.

Drain the onion and put it in a bowl with the celeriac, courgettes, tomatoes and pepper, then stir in the herbs. Whisk all the dressing ingredients together and pour over the vegetables. Stir, then leave to stand for a few minutes before eating. This salad is best served at room temperature.

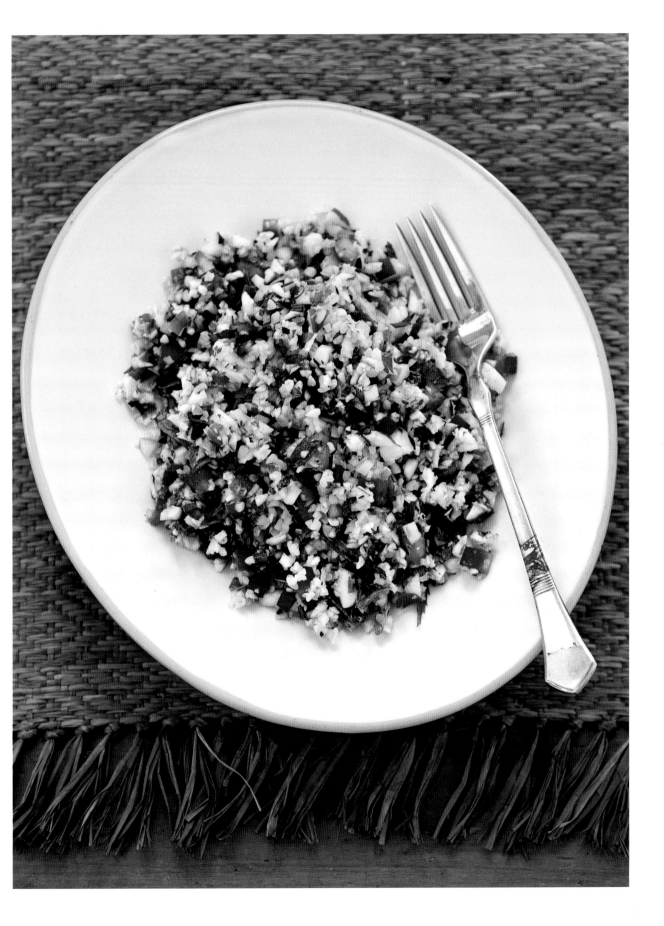

FATTOUSH

163 calories per portion

Eat fattoush for a slim tush! Seriously, though, this is a classic Middle Eastern salad that contains toasted pitta bread to give it a bit more oomph. Sumac, a beautifully tart spice, adds a real punch of flavour and you can find it in most supermarkets now. If you don't have any, the dish will still taste good.

Serves 4
Prep: 15 minutes
Cooking time: 10–15 minutes

2 pitta breads
250g cherry tomatoes, halved
1 large cucumber, diced
2 large or 4 small little gem
    lettuces, cut widthways
    into strips
1 large green pepper, deseeded
    and diced
4 spring onions, sliced into rounds
200g radishes, sliced into rounds
a small bunch of flatleaf parsley,
    finely chopped
a small bunch of mint,
    finely chopped

Dressing
freshly squeezed juice of 1 lemon
1 tbsp olive oil
1 tsp sumac (optional), plus extra
    for sprinkling
pinch of cinnamon
flaked sea salt
freshly ground black pepper

Preheat the oven to 220°C/Fan 200°C/Gas 7.

Cut down the sides of the pitta breads and split them in half so you have 4 thin flatbreads. Put these on a baking tray and bake in the preheated oven until they're crisp and starting to turn golden brown. This should take 10–15 minutes. Remove the pittas from the oven and when they're cool enough to handle – this won't take long at all – tear them into small pieces.

Put the rest of the salad ingredients into a large bowl, add the torn pieces of pitta bread and mix thoroughly.

Whisk together the dressing ingredients and pour the whole lot over the salad. Mix thoroughly with salad spoons or, better still, with your hands.

Serve in large shallow bowls, with a little more sumac sprinkled over the top if you like.

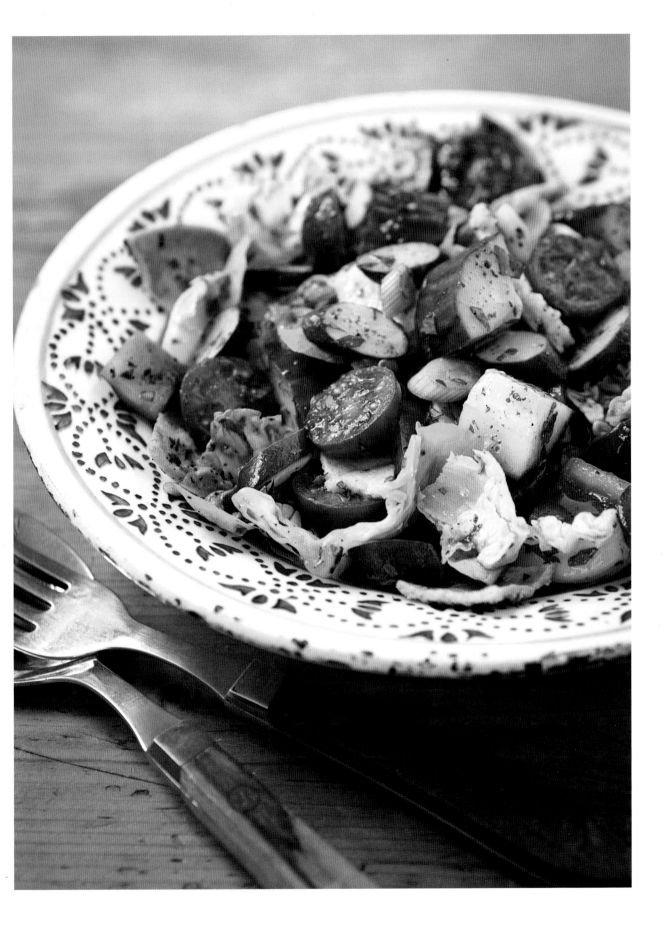

QUINOA SALAD

212 calories per portion

We've been quite bossy about how to put this salad together so you can enjoy it at its fabulous best. If you just mix it all up it will look messy – although it will still be good to eat. If your asparagus is really fresh you can leave it raw for some crunch. Alternatively, you can blanch it briefly or put it on a hot griddle for a few moments for some decorative charring.

Serves 4
Prep: 15 minutes
Cooking time: about 15 minutes

75g quinoa, washed and drained
pinch of salt
8 asparagus spears
2 oranges
100g bag of watercress and spinach
    leaves (or similar)
1 ripe avocado, peeled and cut
    into small chunks
4 spring onions, cut into rounds
leaves from a small bunch of mint

Dressing
1 tbsp olive oil
freshly squeezed juice of 1 lime
1 tbsp soy sauce
½ tsp caster sugar
1 garlic clove, crushed
1 hot red chilli, deseeded and
    finely chopped
flaked sea salt
freshly ground black pepper

To cook the quinoa, tip it into a saucepan with double the volume of water (150ml). Add a pinch of salt and bring to the boil, then cover and turn down the heat. Simmer the quinoa until the water has been absorbed – about 15 minutes. Remove the pan from the heat and leave the quinoa to cool.

Bend each asparagus spear until it snaps and discard the woody end. If you're serving the asparagus raw, simply slice the spears on the diagonal, as thinly as you can, leaving the tips whole. If you prefer your asparagus cooked, blanch or griddle the spears until tender and then slice them thinly.

Peel the oranges and divide them into segments – do this over the bowl you intend making the salad dressing in, so you catch any juice. Set the segments aside and add the rest of the dressing ingredients to the bowl with the juice and whisk them together.

Wash the salad leaves and arrange them on a platter or individual salad plates. Sprinkle over most of the quinoa and spoon over some of the dressing Add the asparagus spears, avocado, orange segments, spring onions and mint leaves. Sprinkle over the rest of the quinoa and pour over the remaining dressing. Toss everything very lightly just before serving.

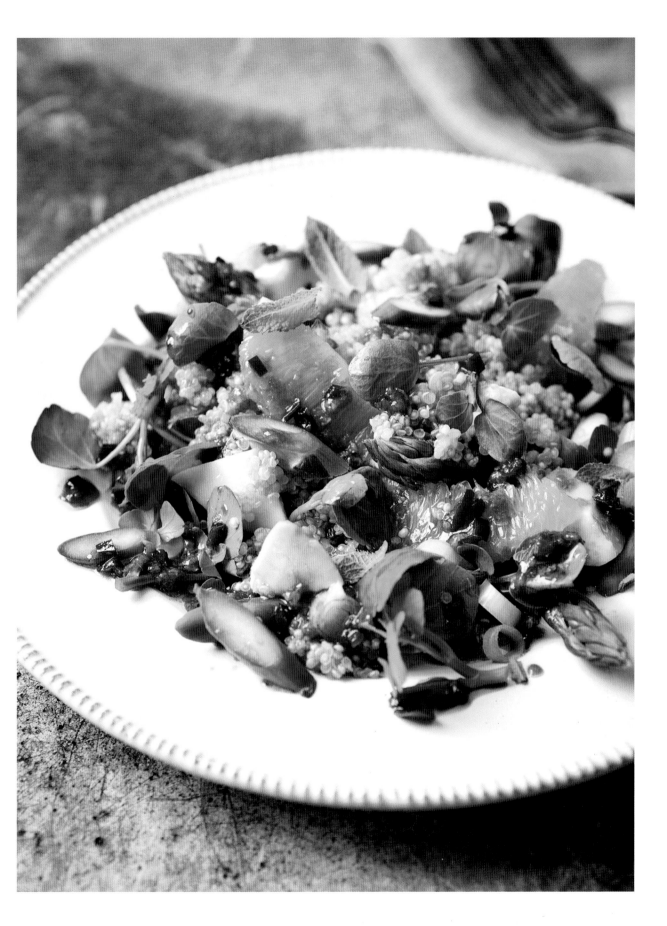

ROOT VEGETABLE BOULANGÈRE

127 calories per portion (if serving 4); 85 calories per portion (if serving 6)

A lovely comforting dish, this was traditionally made just with potatoes and cooked in the baker's oven. Our version uses parsnips and carrots instead of all potatoes to keep the calorie count down and give extra flavour. It's good on its own or goes well with grilled meat.

Serves 4–6
Prep: 10 minutes
Cooking time: about 1 hour

1 large or 2 small parsnips, peeled (about 300g peeled weight)
2 large carrots, peeled (about 250g peeled weight)
2 large potatoes, King Edwards are good (about 400g peeled weight)
oil, for spraying
1 tsp dried sage
2 garlic cloves, finely chopped
600ml vegetable or chicken stock
flaked sea salt
freshly ground black pepper

Preheat the oven to 200°C/Fan 180°C/Gas 6.

Prepare the vegetables. If the parsnips are fat enough, cut them into rounds, otherwise slice into lengths, as thinly as possible. The carrots should also be sliced thinly, but on the diagonal. Finally, cut the potatoes into slightly thicker slices – about 2–3mm.

Spray a baking dish lightly with oil. Arrange the parsnips over the base – you should have enough for at least 2 layers, perhaps 3 if you have managed to slice them very thinly. Follow with half the sage and garlic, then season lightly with salt and pepper.

Add a layer of carrots, then repeat the sage, garlic and seasoning. Finally, top with the potatoes.

Make up the stock with boiling water, or heat gently if using fresh stock, and pour this over the vegetables. Cover the baking dish with a single layer of foil and bake in the preheated oven for half an hour. Uncover the baking dish and cook for another half an hour or until the vegetables are tender and most of the liquid has evaporated.

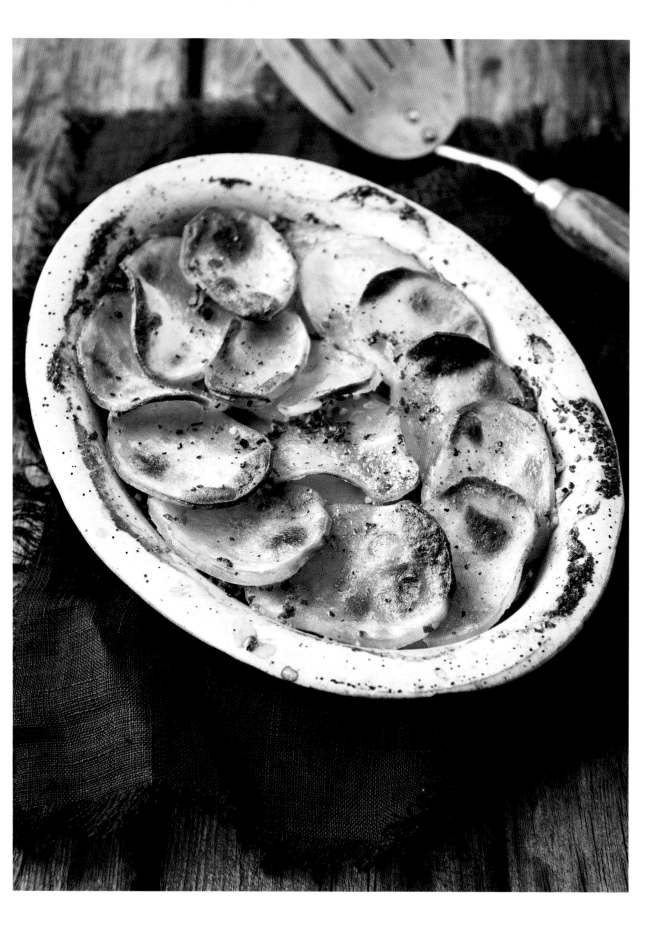

RED CABBAGE WITH APPLE AND CHESTNUTS

76 calories per portion

Serves 8
Prep: 10 minutes
Cooking time: 25–30 minutes

1 tbsp vegetable oil
1 onion, finely chopped
2 garlic cloves, finely chopped
2 eating apples, peeled and grated
　or finely chopped
1 small red cabbage, quartered,
　cored and shredded
a pinch of cinnamon
½ tsp allspice
1 tsp brown sugar
100g vacuum-packed chestnuts,
　roughly chopped
1 tbsp cider vinegar
flaked sea salt
freshly ground black pepper

Many red cabbage recipes need a long cooking time and contain quite a bit of sugar. We've cut down on both here and the result is quick and delicious – and the cabbage keeps its colour. The recipe does make quite a large quantity but freezes brilliantly, so stash some away for another meal if you don't need it all. For a variation, you could use some diced bacon instead of the vinegar and sugar.

Heat the oil in a large saucepan. Add the onion and cook for a few minutes until soft, then add the garlic and cook for another 2 minutes. Now add the apples and cabbage, season with salt and pepper, then sprinkle over the cinnamon, allspice and sugar. Add the chestnuts. Stir the cider vinegar into 100ml of water and pour this into the pan.

Cover and simmer for about 20 minutes until the red cabbage has softened slightly but still has its deep colour.

SPRING GREENS WITH HARISSA AND GARLIC

41 calories per portion

Serves 4
Prep: 5 minutes
Cooking time: 5–8 minutes

1 tsp olive oil
2 garlic cloves, finely chopped
1 tsp–1 tbsp harissa paste, to taste
400g bag of spring greens, washed
　and finely shredded
freshly grated zest of 1 lemon
flaked sea salt
freshly ground black pepper

Make this as hot or not as you like. A teaspoon of harissa gives a mellow heat while a tablespoon packs more of a punch – up to you.

Heat the olive oil in a large frying pan or saucepan with a lid. Add the garlic cloves and harissa paste and cook for a couple of minutes, stirring constantly.

Add 100ml of water and stir to combine with the garlic and paste, then add the greens. Turn the greens over so they are coated with the sauce, then season with salt and pepper. Cover and cook on a medium heat for about 5 minutes, stirring every so often, until the spring greens have wilted, but still have a little bite to them. Add the lemon zest at the last minute.

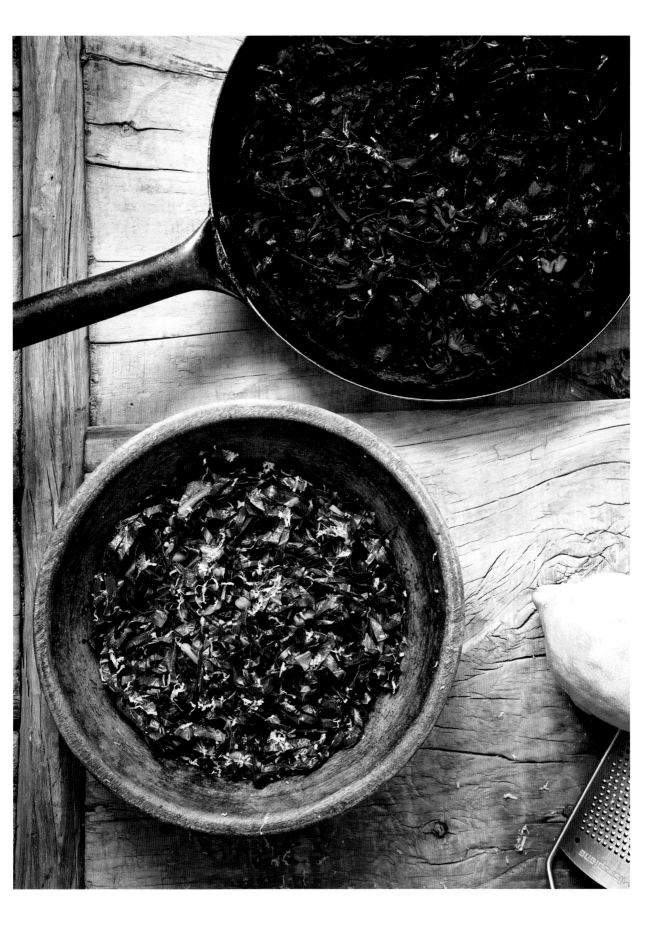

GREEK-STYLE ROAST VEGETABLES

176 calories per portion (if serving 4); 117 calories per portion (if serving 6)

This kind of one-pot vegetable dish usually contains loads of olive oil and so is high in calories. We've found that you can get away with just a small amount of oil and loads of juicy veg and it still tastes fantastic. The veg are good cold too, so make extra and use in a salad.

Serves 4–6
Prep: 15 minutes
Cooking time: 1 hour

300g potatoes, unpeeled and sliced into rounds
2 large courgettes, sliced into rounds
2 red onions, peeled and cut into thin wedges
2 peppers (red or green) cut into chunks
a few garlic cloves, unpeeled
1 tsp dried oregano or mixed herbs
1 tbsp olive oil
100ml white wine
300ml vegetable stock, chicken stock or water
12 cherry tomatoes
flaked sea salt
freshly ground black pepper

Preheat the oven to 200°C/Fan 180°C/Gas 6.

Put all the vegetables and garlic in a large roasting tin or shallow casserole dish. Sprinkle over the herbs and season well with salt and pepper. Drizzle over the olive oil, then mix everything together with your hands so all the vegetables have a coating of oil.

Mix the wine and stock or water and pour over the vegetables. Either cover your roasting tin with foil or put the lid on your casserole dish, then place in the preheated oven for half an hour.

Remove the foil or lid and gently turn everything over with a spoon. Dot the cherry tomatoes around the dish, then put it back in the oven for another half an hour, uncovered, until most of the liquid has evaporated and the vegetables have started to brown.

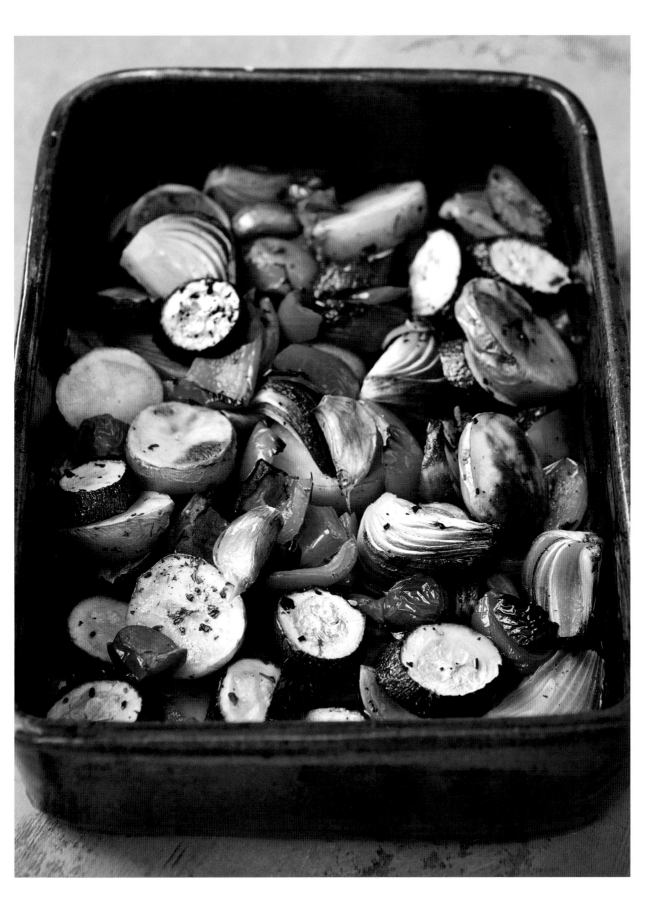

ROASTED CARROT, PEPPER AND CHICKPEA SALAD

136 calories per portion

You can make the zingy dressing for this salad with orange or lemon, but we like to add a pinch of caster sugar or a little drizzle of honey if using lemon. With orange, add a tiny squeeze of lemon juice. The salad can be served on its own with some leaves or to accompany some plain grilled meat.

Serves 4
Prep: 20 minutes
Cooking time: 35 minutes

2 large carrots, peeled and cut
    into 2cm chunks
1 tsp ground cumin
1 tsp olive oil
2 red peppers, deseeded and cut
    in half, lengthways
400g can of chickpeas, drained
    and rinsed
2 tbsp chopped dill
2 tbsp chopped mint
2 tbsp chopped parsley or coriander
flaked sea salt
freshly ground black pepper

Dressing
1 tsp tahini
1 tsp olive oil
freshly squeezed juice of 1 orange
    or lemon
1 garlic clove, crushed
¼ tsp allspice
½ tsp cumin
pinch of caster sugar or small
    drizzle of honey (optional)

Preheat the oven to 220°C/Fan 200°C/Gas 7. Line a roasting dish with baking parchment.

Bring a saucepan of water to the boil. Add a pinch of salt and the carrots and simmer for 15 minutes until they're almost tender. Drain the carrots and tip them into the roasting dish, then season with salt, pepper and cumin. Drizzle with the olive oil.

Push the carrots into one half of the roasting dish and put the peppers in the other half, cut side down. Roast for 20 minutes until the carrots have taken on some colour and the peppers are starting to soften and look slightly charred. Remove the dish from the oven and put the peppers in a bag or a covered bowl and leave them to steam until they are cool enough to handle. Peel off the skin – it should come off easily – and cut or tear the peppers into thin strips.

To make the dressing, whisk all the ingredients together and season with salt and pepper. If using lemon juice, you might like to add a pinch of caster sugar or a little drizzle of honey.

To assemble the salad, put the carrots, peppers and chickpeas in a large bowl. Add all the herbs, then pour over the dressing. Mix everything together, then leave to stand at room temperature for a while to let the flavours develop before serving.

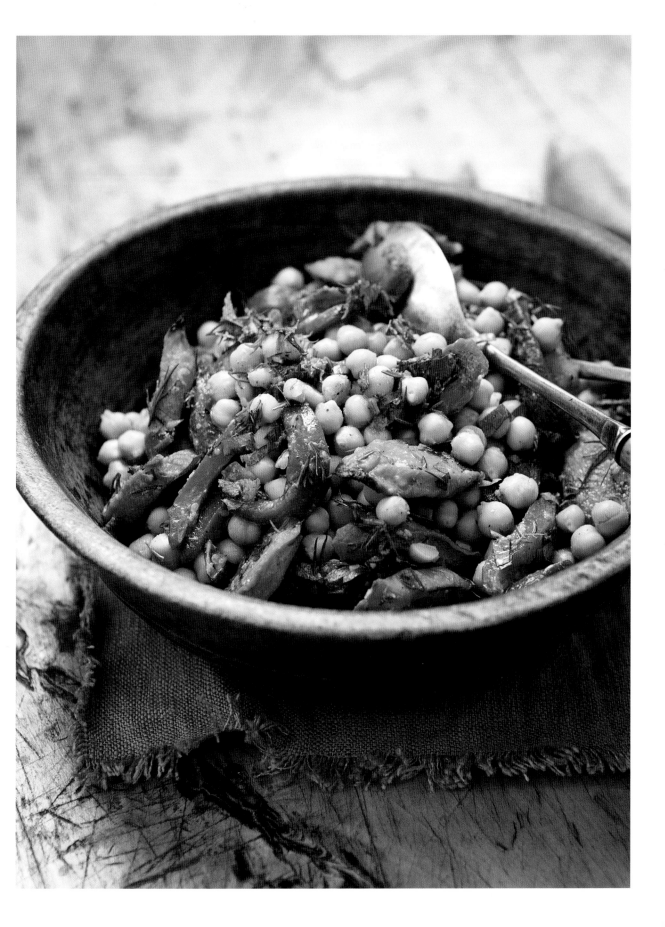

SUNSHINE FOOD

We both love Mediterranean-style and Middle Eastern food, with all those great flavours of herbs, spices and wonderful veg. And, of course, we discovered that if you cut down on the oil a bit, these sunshine dishes can be healthy, low-cal eating as well as good eating. Try our recipes for Italian ribollita and Moroccan harira soups – both a meal in themselves. Or cook up some souvlaki or lamb burgers and tzatziki, put your sunnies on and imagine yourself on a terrace overlooking the Med – maybe even in that new swimsuit you can now wear with pride!

BEAN AND VEGETABLE SOUP

290 calories per portion

Our version of ribollita, a classic Italian recipe, this is a good hearty soup. We've used less pasta than usual, but there are plenty of beans and veg. Use any sort of cabbage you like, including spring greens, kale or Swiss chard, but don't be tempted to try spinach – it will just end up as mush. This is also a great recipe for using up a bit of Parmesan rind if you have one in the fridge – provides some extra punch and flavour.

Serves 4
Prep: 15 minutes
Cooking time: about 40 minutes

1 tbsp olive oil
50g back bacon, trimmed of fat
   and finely diced
1 onion, finely chopped
1 fennel bulb, trimmed and
   finely chopped
2 carrots, finely chopped
2 celery sticks, chopped
4 garlic cloves, finely chopped
1 tsp dried oregano
a Parmesan rind (optional)
100ml red wine
400g can of cannellini beans,
   drained and rinsed
4 fresh tomatoes, finely chopped, or
   200g canned chopped tomatoes
600ml chicken stock
50g pasta (any short form will do)
½ green cabbage or the equivalent
   in other greens
1 large courgette, diagonally sliced
squeeze of lemon juice (optional)
flaked sea salt
freshly ground black pepper

To serve
handful of basil leaves, roughly torn
25g Parmesan cheese, grated

Heat the olive oil in a large saucepan or casserole dish. Add the diced bacon and fry until crisp and brown. Add the onion, fennel, carrots, celery and garlic and sauté for a couple of minutes. Sprinkle over the oregano, add the Parmesan rind, if using, then pour over the red wine. Bring to the boil and simmer until the wine has reduced by about half.

Add the beans and tomatoes, then pour in the stock. Bring the soup back to the boil and simmer for about 15 minutes until all the vegetables are tender. Add the pasta and cabbage, continue to simmer for 5 minutes, then add the courgette. Simmer for another 5–10 minutes until the pasta is cooked al dente and all the vegetables are cooked through. Check for seasoning and if you think the soup needs it, add a squeeze of lemon juice.

Sprinkle over the basil and serve with a scant tablespoon each of grated Parmesan.

FREEZE!

This freezes well but best to add the courgette after defrosting.

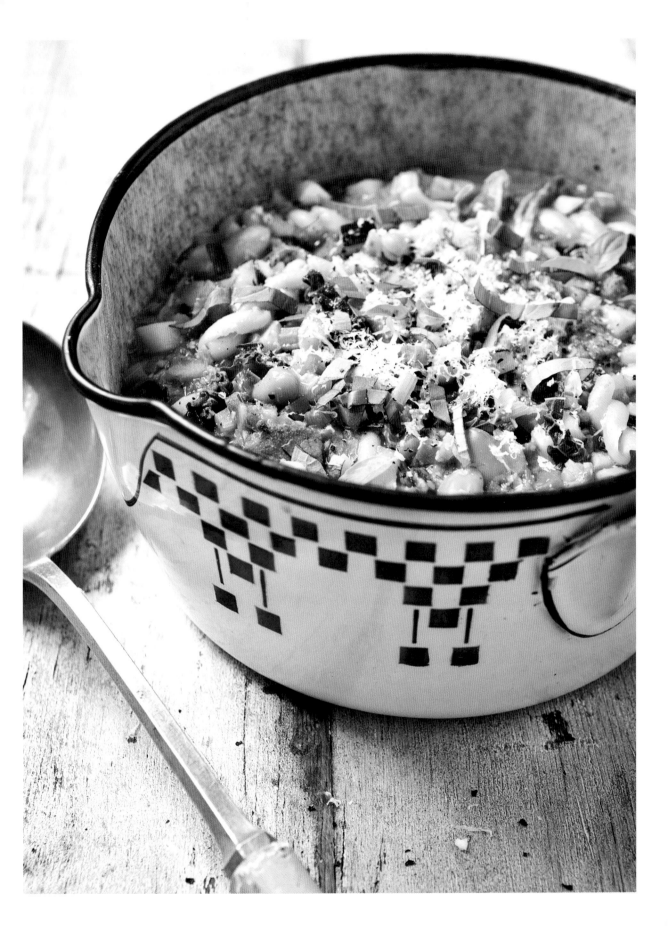

SPICY MOROCCAN SOUP

330 calories per portion (if serving 4); 220 calories per portion (if serving 6)

This is our quick way of making a Moroccan soup known as harira, which is the traditional way to break your fast at Ramadan. It's fragrant, spicy and very nourishing and doesn't take long to make. If you don't have all the spices you could use a spice blend such as ras-el-hanout or harissa instead. Both are available in supermarkets.

Serves 4–6
Prep: 15 minutes
Cooking time: 1 hour 15 minutes

1 tbsp olive oil
2 onions, sliced
2 peppers (1 red, 1 green), deseeded and cut into strips
250g lamb, preferably leg meat, finely diced into ½–1cm cubes
1 tsp turmeric
1 tsp ground ginger
1 tsp ground coriander
2 tsp ground cumin
½ tsp cinnamon
½ tsp hot chilli powder
1 pinch of saffron strands
1 garlic clove
1 litre chicken stock or water
400g can of tomatoes
2 tbsp chopped fresh coriander, plus extra for serving
2 tbsp chopped flatleaf parsley, plus extra for serving
400g can of chickpeas, drained and rinsed
50g long-grain rice
freshly squeezed juice of ½ lemon
flaked sea salt
freshly ground black pepper

Heat the olive oil in a large saucepan. Add the onions and peppers and cook for a few minutes over a low to medium heat until they start to soften. Turn up the heat, add the lamb and brown it quickly on all sides.

Turn the heat down again and add all the spices (or the spice blend, if using) and the garlic. Sauté for a couple more minutes until everything is well combined, then pour in the stock. Season with salt and freshly ground black pepper. Bring to the boil, then turn the heat down and leave the soup to simmer for 30 minutes.

Put the tomatoes in a blender with 2 tablespoons each of coriander and parsley and blitz until the herbs are very finely chopped. Pour this mixture into the saucepan, then add the chickpeas and rice. Simmer for another 30 minutes, by which time the meat should be beautifully tender.

Just before serving, stir in the lemon juice and taste for seasoning, then adjust if necessary. Sprinkle with extra chopped coriander and parsley and serve.

FREEZE!

Freezes very well. It's best to add the lemon juice after defrosting as certain flavours – garlic and ginger in particular – intensify on freezing and you might not need it. Taste first and add lemon if you think it's necessary.

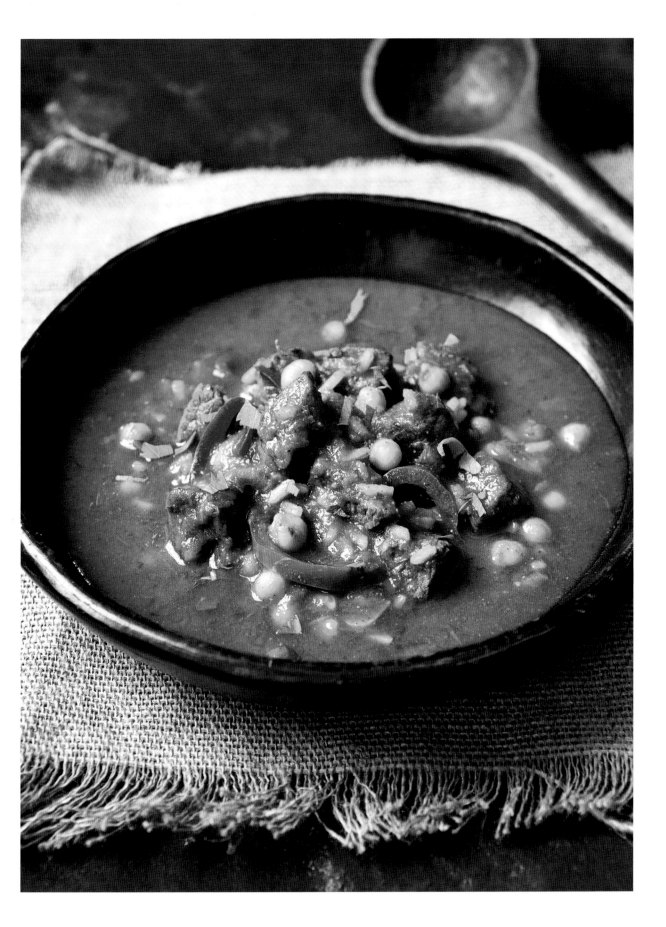

MACKEREL FILLETS WITH GREMOLATA

339 calories per portion;

Gremolata is the name for a simple but tasty Italian garnish. It's just finely chopped garlic, parsley and lemon zest but it adds a fantastic zingy flavour to chicken, meat or fish, such as this super-speedy mackerel dish. We've suggested cooking the fish in a frying pan with just a light spritz of oil, but you could also do it on a griddle or a barbecue – with one of those fish cages. Lovely served with a tomato and onion salad if you fancy.

Serves 2
Prep: 10 minutes
Cooking time: 5 minutes

oil, for spraying
4 small mackerel fillets,
    about 300g in total
2 tbsp finely chopped flatleaf
    parsley
2 garlic cloves, finely chopped
finely grated zest of 1 lemon
flaked sea salt
freshly ground black pepper

Tomato and onion salad
1 small sweet white onion, finely
    sliced into crescents
2 or 3 very ripe vine tomatoes
1 tsp olive oil
squeeze of lemon juice
a pinch of sugar
1 tbsp finely chopped flatleaf
    parsley
1 tsp salted capers, rinsed (optional)
flaked sea salt
finely ground white pepper

Lightly spray a large non-stick frying pan with oil and place it over a medium heat. Season the mackerel fillets with salt and pepper. Put the fillets in the pan, skin-side down, and cook for 3–4 minutes. When the flesh of the mackerel is almost completely white and opaque, turn the fillets over and cook for another minute.

Mix the parsley, garlic and lemon zest together to make the gremolata. Serve the mackerel with the gremolata on the side, for sprinkling over.

Tomato and onion salad
Soaking onions before using them raw takes off that really astringent edge. But again, if you don't mind that, you can leave out the soaking step.

Sprinkle salt over the onion slices and put them in a bowl of very cold water. Leave for 10 minutes, then drain. Slice the tomatoes horizontally into thin rounds and arrange them on a plate. Sprinkle over the onion crescents.

Whisk together the olive oil, lemon juice, sugar, salt and white pepper. Pour this over the tomatoes and onions. Sprinkle over the parsley and the capers, if using. Leave for a few minutes to allow the flavours to develop, then serve at room temperature.

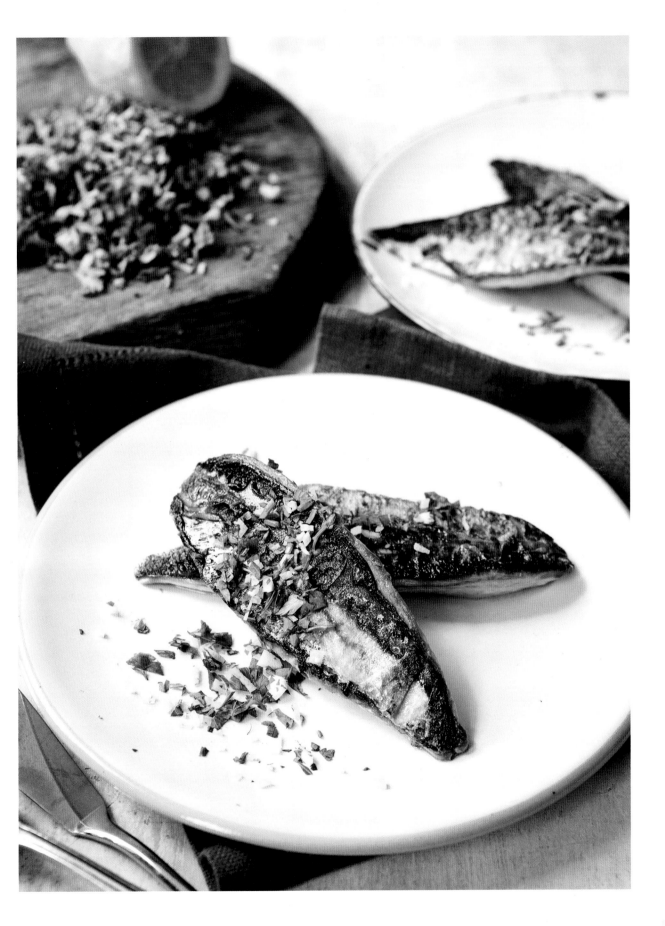

CHICKEN CACCIATORE

281 calories per portion

This is an old-fashioned dish but one that's very popular with the 18–30s – we mean age here, not dress size. It's great just as it is but you can also add some thinly sliced veg, such as red peppers and celery, if you like.

Serves 4
Prep: 15 minutes
Cooking time: about 1 hour
15 minutes

1 tbsp olive oil
2 onions, finely sliced
4 garlic cloves, finely chopped
a large sprig of rosemary
4 bone-in chicken thighs, skinned,
4 chicken drumsticks, skinned
150ml white wine
150ml chicken stock
200g fresh tomatoes, peeled and
   deseeded and chopped, or 200g
   canned chopped tomatoes
handful of flatleaf parsley, chopped
flaked sea salt
freshly ground black pepper

Heat the olive oil in a large casserole dish on the hob. Add the onions and cook them over a low heat until they are soft and translucent – this should take about 15 minutes. Add the garlic and rosemary and cook for another couple of minutes.

Turn the heat up, push the onions to one side and add the chicken pieces. Fry them, turning the pieces over once or twice until they are very lightly browned, then mix with the onions.

Pour in the white wine and allow it to bubble down. Add the chicken stock and tomatoes, then season with salt and pepper. Turn the heat down, cover the dish and leave to simmer gently for about 45 minutes until the chicken is cooked through and very tender. Sprinkle with chopped parsley and serve with some green veg.

FREEZE!

This freezes well. To use, defrost thoroughly and reheat gently, adding a little more liquid if necessary. Stir as little as possible while reheating so you don't break up the chicken too much.

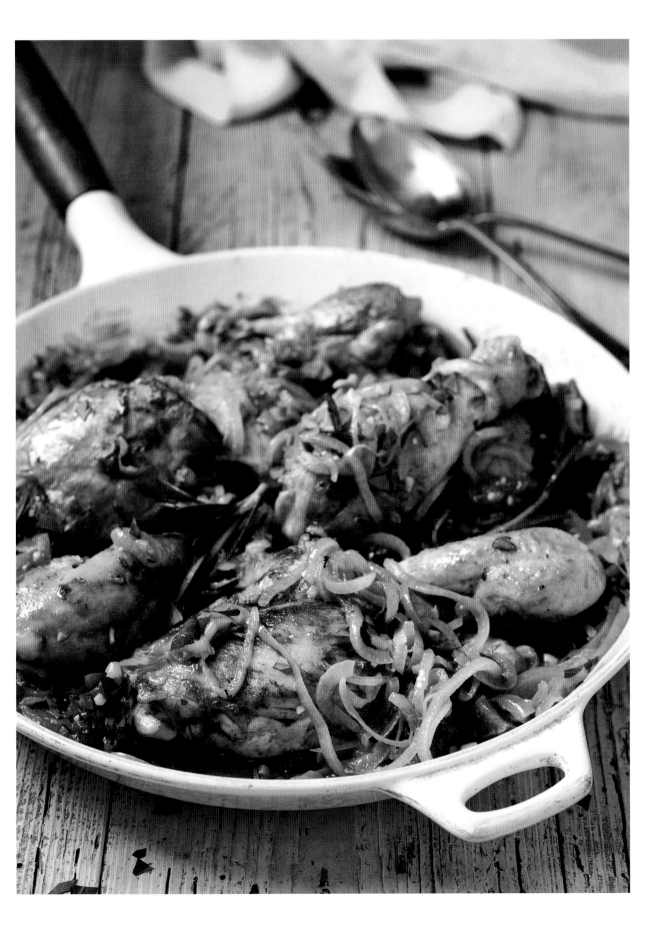

LAMB BURGERS WITH TZATZIKI

385 calories per portion (if serving 4);
257 calories per portion (if serving 6)

Flavoured with chopped herbs and lemon zest, these burgers have a real Mediterranean zing.

Serves 4–6
Prep: 20 minutes
Cooking time: 12–15 minutes

1 tsp olive oil
1 onion, finely chopped
2 garlic cloves, finely chopped
500g lean lamb mince
50g breadcrumbs
2 tsp dried mint
1 tsp dried oregano
1 tsp finely chopped rosemary
zest of 1 lemon
small pinch of cinnamon
50g low-fat natural yoghurt
flaked sea salt
freshly ground black pepper

Tzatziki
1 large cucumber
250g low-fat natural yoghurt
2 garlic cloves, crushed
1 tsp white wine vinegar
2 tsp dried mint

FREEZE!

The burgers/balls freeze well, raw or cooked. Open freeze them on a baking tray, then when solid, put in bags to store. Don't try to freeze the tzatziki!

Preheat the oven to 220°C/Fan 200°C/Gas 7. Line a baking tray with baking parchment.

Heat the oil in a frying pan. Add the chopped onion and cook, stirring regularly, until it's soft and translucent. Add the garlic cloves and cook for another 2 minutes. Remove the pan from the heat and allow the onion and garlic to cool.

Put the lamb in a bowl and break up any clumps. Season generously with salt and pepper and sprinkle over the breadcrumbs, herbs, lemon zest and cinnamon. Add the onions and garlic, along with the yoghurt, and mix the whole lot together. The easiest way to do this is with your hands. Divide the mixture into 6 portions and form burger-sized patties. Alternatively, if you prefer meatballs, shape them into balls the size of a golf ball – about 40g each.

Space the burgers or balls on the baking tray. Bake them in the oven for 12–15 minutes, until well browned. If you want the lamb slightly pink in the middle, cook for 10 minutes. Serve with tzatziki.

Tzatziki

Peel the cucumber and cut it in half lengthways. Scoop out the seeds with a teaspoon and discard. Coarsely grate the cucumber and put it in a colander. Sprinkle it with salt and leave over a bowl or in the sink to drain for half an hour.

After half an hour, wring out as much water from the cucumber as you can. A good way to do this is to put it all on a clean tea towel, scrunch the tea towel up into a bundle and twist the edges together, then squeeze hard! You'll be amazed at how much water comes out. Put the yoghurt in a bowl and add the garlic, white wine vinegar and mint. Add the cucumber and stir well.

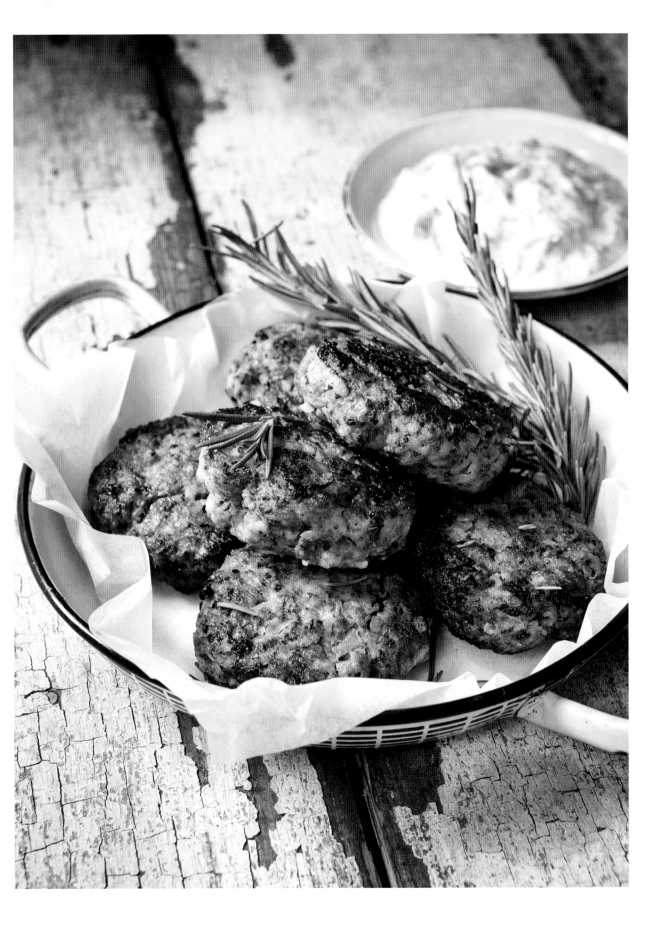

PORK SOUVLAKI WITH LIGHT SALSA VERDE

270 calories per portion (if serving 4);
180 calories per portion (if serving 6)

These pork kebabs are satisfaction on a stick. Salsa verde goes beautifully with them but usually contains shedloads of olive oil. We've come up with something that's more like a herby mayonnaise and we really love it – see what you think.

Serves 4–6
Prep: 15 minutes,
plus marinating
Cooking time: 12–15 minutes

700g lean pork, diced into
   3cm chunks

Marinade
1 tsp olive oil
juice of 1 lemon
1 tsp dried mint
1 tsp dried oregano
1 bay leaf, crumbled
1 tbsp red wine vinegar
flaked sea salt
freshly ground black pepper

Light salsa verde
1 egg yolk
1 heaped tsp Dijon mustard
1 tbsp olive oil
juice of 1 lemon
2 anchovies, finely chopped
   (optional)
2 tbsp capers, rinsed and chopped
a large bunch of flatleaf parsley
   leaves, finely chopped
a small bunch of basil, finely
   chopped
a small bunch of mint, finely
   chopped
flaked sea salt
freshly ground black pepper

Mix all the marinade ingredients together in a large non-metallic bowl. Add the pork and stir until it's all completely covered, then leave to marinate in the fridge for at least half an hour – it's fine to leave it overnight if that suits you.

If you're using bamboo skewers, soak them in water for half an hour before you need them – this will prevent them from burning. Thread the pork chunks on to 8 skewers. Cook the souvlaki on a hot barbecue, on a griddle pan on the hob (you may have to do this in batches) or under a hot grill, for 12–15 minutes. Turn the skewers regularly, until all the meat is charred and cooked through.

Serve the pork kebabs on or off the skewers, with the sauce on the side; nice with a simple tomato and onion salad (see page 144).

Light salsa verde
Put the egg yolk in a bowl with the mustard. Whisk them together, then add the olive oil, a few drops at a time so the mixture emulsifies properly. Whisk in the lemon juice, then stir in all the remaining ingredients. If you want a very smooth sauce, blitz it briefly in a blender. You can also add a tablespoon of water if you prefer the sauce slightly thinner.

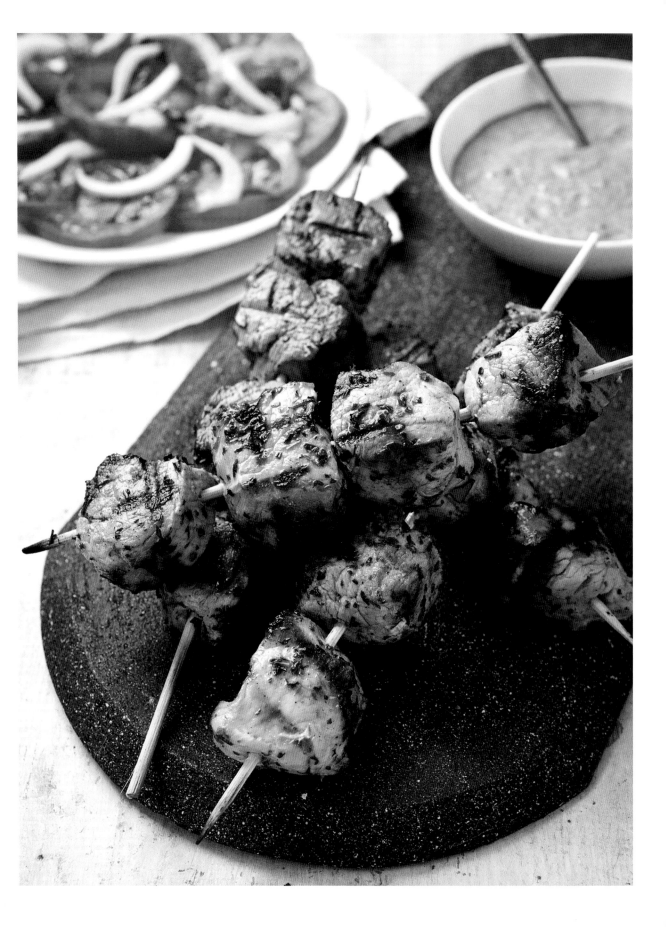

PORK SALTIMBOCCA

194 calories per portion

We watched Antonio Carluccio cook this fab Italian dish and couldn't wait to try it ourselves. It usually contains quite a bit of butter, but we've taken that out and kept the lovely tasty ham and sage so it's really good to eat. You can reduce the calorie count by removing the fat from the ham, but we like to leave it on for extra flavour.

Serves 4
Prep: 15 minutes
Cooking time: about 10 minutes

4 small medallions of pork fillet
    or loin, about 100g each
4 slices of Parma ham
2 tsp dried sage
finely grated zest of 1 lemon
2 tsp olive oil
100ml Marsala wine (or you could
    use medium sherry)
50ml chicken stock or water
squeeze of lemon juice
freshly ground black pepper

Put a pork medallion between 2 large sheets of cling film. Flatten it with a rolling pin or the smooth side of a meat mallet until you have a very thin escalope – about ½ cm. Repeat with the remaining pieces of pork.

Sprinkle each escalope with dried sage and lemon zest, then season with pepper – not salt, as the ham is salty enough. Top with a slice of Parma ham and press it down firmly. If any edges of the ham overlap the pork, just tuck them underneath.

Heat 1 teaspoon of the olive oil in a large frying pan. Fry 2 of the pork escalopes at a time – they will only need 2 minutes on each side. You should find that the Parma ham will stick to the escalope without any problem. Transfer the escalopes to a plate and keep them warm while you cook the rest. If the frying pan seems a bit dry, add the second teaspoon of olive oil.

Pour the Marsala into the frying pan and allow it to bubble up while you scrape any sticky bits off the bottom of the pan, then add the water or stock. Simmer for a couple of minutes to reduce – you want a sauce with the consistency of a very light syrup. Drain off any juice that may have come from the resting escalopes and add this to the sauce, together with a squeeze of lemon juice. Serve the escalopes with the sauce spooned over and perhaps a salad, such as our fattoush (see page 126).

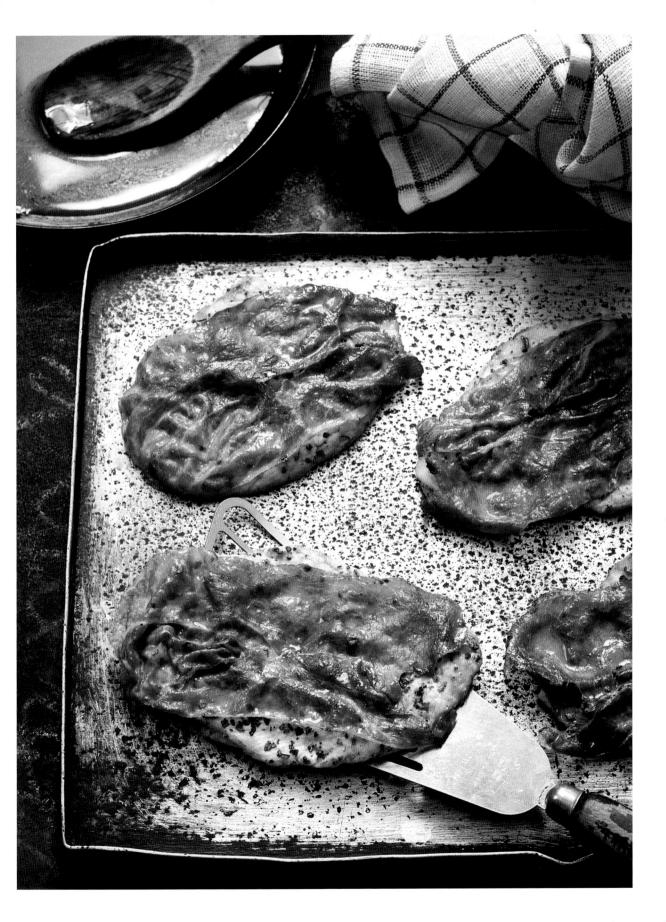

SANDWICHES, DIPS AND SNACKS

Diet or no diet, we all need a quick satisfying snack from time to time and we're constantly asked what we do about food on the move. It's true that we have to think a bit to stay out of trouble but we're getting better at it. Our latest dip recipes can be eaten straight from the fridge with crunchy veg sticks when you come home starving, or made into open sandwiches or wraps for a light meal or to pop in your lunch box. The pad Thai omelette was inspired by the street food we enjoyed in Thailand and the cauliflower nuggets taste like a naughty bar snack but come in at under 100 calories a portion. Can't say fairer than that.

POTATO BREAD

about 65 calories per slice, cut into 20 slices

We first came across potato bread in Germany when we were working on our
Big Book of Baking. You might be surprised to hear this, but replacing some
of the flour in bread with mashed potato cuts the calories! Strange but true.
You'll love this bread and it's brilliant for sandwiches.

Makes 1 loaf
Prep: 25 minutes, plus proving time
Cooking time: 30 minutes

375g potatoes, preferably Maris
   Pipers or King Edwards
oil, for spraying
1 sachet (about 7g) of fast-acting
   dried yeast
1 tsp sugar
1 tsp salt
300g strong white flour
75ml warm water

FREEZE!

Freezes well. You can slice
the loaf before freezing –
should get about 20 slices
– and then take them out
of the freezer as you need.
The bread is best toasted
after freezing.

First, make the mash so it can cool down before you use it. Peel the potatoes and cut them into chunks of about 3cm. Put them in a large saucepan, cover with cold water and bring to the boil. Cook for 10–15 minutes or until very tender – test them with the tip of a knife. Drain the potatoes in a large colander and tip them back into the saucepan, then mash until smooth – don't add any butter or milk. Leave the mash to cool but it doesn't have to be stone cold before using. Lightly spray a 2lb loaf tin with oil.

Put 300g of the mashed potato in a large bowl and sprinkle over the yeast and sugar. Give it a quick mix so the yeast isn't all on the surface of the potato, then add the salt. Add the flour, then gradually mix in the water until you have a fairly tacky dough.

Turn the dough out on to a lightly floured work surface and knead for a few minutes until soft and pliable. Put it back in the bowl, cover it with a damp tea towel and leave it somewhere warm to rise for about an hour. When the dough has doubled in size, knock it back and turn it out on to the work surface again. Knead it into a loaf shape, tucking the edges under so you have a smooth, domed oblong. Put the dough in a loaf tin, cover again and leave to rise. Preheat the oven to its highest setting.

After about half an hour the bread should have risen well in its tin. Put it in the oven and immediately turn the temperature down to 220°C/Fan 200°C/Gas 7. Bake for about 30 minutes until the crust is firm and a deep golden brown and the base sounds hollow when you knock on it. Turn the loaf out on to a wire rack and leave to cool before using.

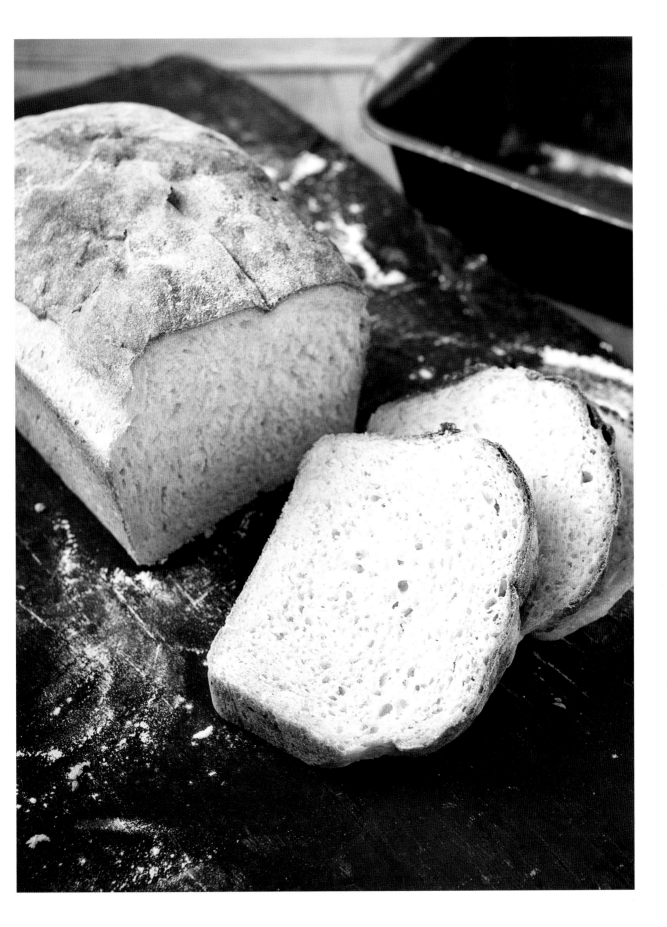

MIXED GRAIN BREAD FOR OPEN SANDWICHES

85 calories per thin slice

A slightly dense, filling loaf, this is good for slicing thinly and toasting or using as is for open sandwiches. It won't rise as much as an all-wheat loaf, but it is easy to make and tastes great. Using a starter mixture improves the taste and texture of the bread, but you do need to prepare that the day before.

Makes 1 loaf
Prep: 25 minutes, plus proving time and starter fermentation
Cooking time: 30 minutes

Starter
100g strong white bread flour
125ml water
2g dried yeast (small pinch)

Dough
starter mix (see above)
150g white bread flour
100g wholemeal flour
150g rye flour
175ml water
5g dried yeast
1 tsp salt
1 tsp honey

oil, for spraying the tin

To make the starter mixture, put the ingredients in a bowl and mix them together – the mixture will be the consistency of a very sloppy dough or paste. Cover and leave at room temperature overnight or for at least 16 hours. You can leave the starter for a couple of days if you like, but your bread will taste much stronger.

To make the bread, put the starter into a large bowl (or the bowl of a food mixer) and add all the other ingredients. Mix until firm, then knead until you have a smooth dough. This will take at least 5 minutes with the dough hook on a food mixer, longer if kneading by hand. Then spend a couple of minutes stretching the dough away from you as far as possible and folding it back to you – this will help develop a chewy texture and introduce air bubbles into the dough.

Put the dough in a bowl and cover with a damp tea towel. Leave for at least an hour, preferably 2, until the dough is well risen. Lightly spray a 2lb loaf tin with oil.

Knock the dough back, shape it into a long oblong and put it into the tin. Cover again and leave for another 30–60 minutes. At this point, preheat the oven to its highest setting. If you put the bread on top of the oven, the residual heat will help with the proving.

When the dough has risen again and feels springy to the touch, put it in the oven. Immediately reduce the temperature to 220°C/Fan 200°C/Gas 7 and bake for about 30 minutes until a dark golden brown crust has formed and the bread sounds hollow when tapped on the bottom. Leave to cool on a wire rack.

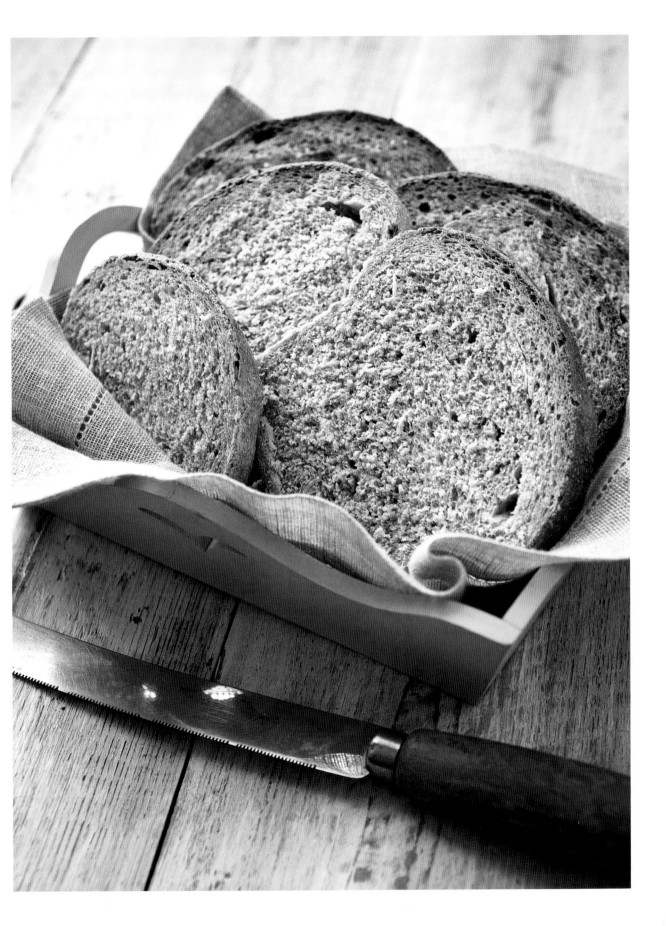

Makes 4 portions of dip, 4 open sandwiches or 2 wraps

150g smoked trout fillets
2 tbsp low-fat crème fraiche
1 tsp horseradish sauce
¼ cucumber, peeled, deseeded and chopped
1 tbsp finely chopped dill
squeeze of lemon juice
flaked sea salt
freshly ground black pepper

Open sandwiches
2 cooked beetroot, thinly sliced
4 slices of firm bread, such as rye
a few sprigs of dill

Wraps
2 large tortilla wraps
bunch of watercress
2 cooked beetroot, finely sliced

SMOKED TROUT DIP OR FILLING

58 calories per portion (dip); 146 calories per open sandwich; 157 calories per wrap

Break the trout into small pieces, removing any bones, and put them in a bowl. In another bowl, mix the crème fraiche and horseradish. Add the cucumber and dill to the trout, then fold in the crème fraiche and horseradish mixture. Taste and season with salt and pepper and, if you think it needs it, a squeeze of lemon juice. If you are having this as a dip, purée or mash until it is quite smooth and serve with sticks of carrot, celery and cucumber.

To make open sandwiches, put a layer of beetroot on slices of bread and top with the trout. Garnish with a few sprigs of dill.

To make wraps, cover each tortilla wrap with sprigs of watercress, then follow with the beetroot. Pile the trout on top. Fold up the bottom of each wrap to stop everything falling out, then roll the whole thing up tightly. Cut in half on the diagonal. If you are not using immediately, wrap in foil or baking parchment for later.

Makes 4 portions of dip, 4 open sandwiches or 2 wraps

1 can of tuna in spring water
juice of 1 lime
2 tbsp light mayonnaise
1 tbsp low-fat crème fraiche
a dash of Tabasco
1 tbsp capers, chopped
¼ red pepper, finely chopped
2 spring onions, finely chopped
2 tbsp coriander, finely chopped

Open sandwiches
4 slices of bread
¼ cucumber
pinch of sugar
1 tsp white wine vinegar

Wraps
2 large wraps
2 large lettuce leaves, shredded
¼ cucumber, finely sliced lengthways
a handful of mint

TUNA AND CAPER DIP OR FILLING

61 calories per portion (dip); 118 calories per open sandwich; 236 calories per wrap

Drain the tuna and put it in a food processor with the lime juice, mayonnaise and crème fraiche and blitz until smooth. Stir in the rest of the ingredients and check for seasoning. Serve as a dip with sticks of carrot and cucumber or pile into lettuce leaves.

To make open sandwiches, slice the cucumber as thinly as you can. Dissolve a pinch of sugar in the vinegar and a tablespoon of water and pour this over the cucumber. Toss it lightly, then drain. Put the slices of cucumber on the bread and top with the tuna.

To make wraps, cover each wrap with lettuce, then follow with cucumber. Put the tuna mix on top, then add the mint. Fold up the bottom of each wrap to stop everything falling out, then roll the whole thing up tightly. Cut in half on the diagonal. If you are not using immediately, wrap in foil or baking parchment for later.

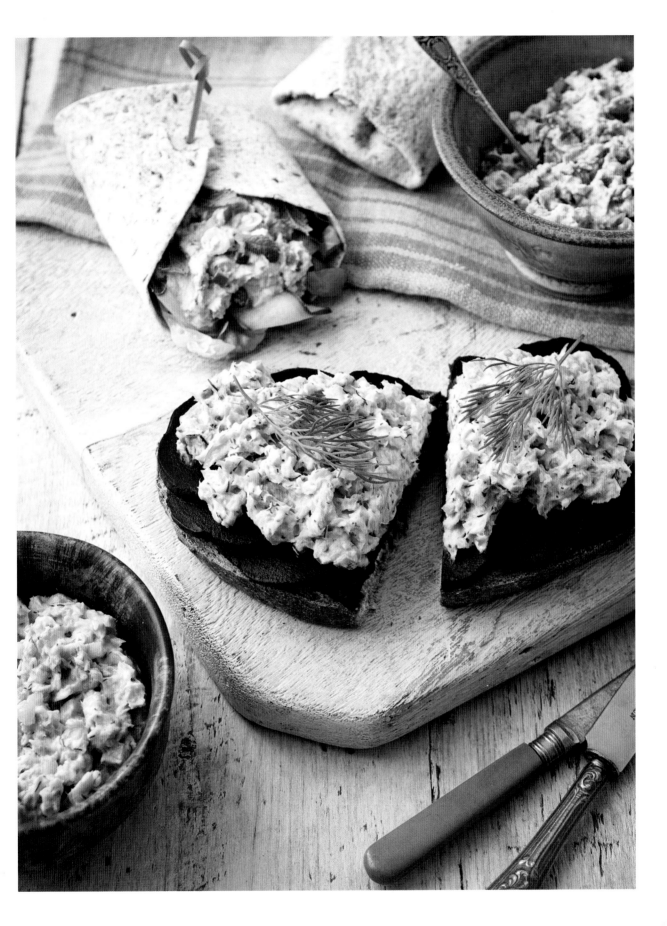

CARROT, RED PEPPER AND BUTTERBEAN DIP

64 calories per portion

You could use chickpeas or any other kind of bean for this but butterbeans do work well. There's very little oil in the dip, which saves on calories, but the crème fraiche or yoghurt really improves the texture and gives great mouth feel. Serve with some radishes and sticks of crunchy carrot, cucumber and celery.

Serves 8
Prep: 10 minutes
Cooking time: 35 minutes

2 large carrots, peeled and cut
    into rounds
1 head of garlic, broken into cloves
    and left unpeeled (2 cloves
    reserved)
1 large red pepper, deseeded
    and halved
1 tsp olive oil
400g can of butterbeans, drained
    and rinsed
1 tsp cumin
½ tsp sweet smoked paprika
¼ tsp cayenne or chilli powder
1 tsp tahini
2 tbsp low-fat crème fraiche
    or yoghurt
squeeze of lemon juice (optional)
flaked sea salt
freshly ground black pepper

To serve
1 tsp olive oil
extra paprika and cayenne

Preheat the oven to its highest temperature. Bring a saucepan of water to the boil and add the carrots and garlic – having set aside 2 of the cloves. Simmer for 15 minutes, then drain thoroughly and spread them over half of a roasting tin. Put the red pepper in the other half of the tin. Drizzle over the olive oil, then put the veg in the oven and roast for 20 minutes, until the carrots have started to take on colour and the red pepper is soft.

Put the red pepper in a bag or a covered bowl and set aside. When it is cool enough to handle, peel off the skin. Squeeze the flesh out of the garlic cloves and put this in a food processor with the red pepper, carrots, butterbeans, cumin, paprika, cayenne or chilli powder and the tahini. Finely chop the reserved garlic cloves and add those too. Season with salt and pepper.

Purée the dip until smooth, then fold in the crème fraiche. Taste for seasoning and add a squeeze of lemon juice if you like.

Scoop the dip into a bowl and serve drizzled with a teaspoon of oil and sprinkled with a little paprika and cayenne.

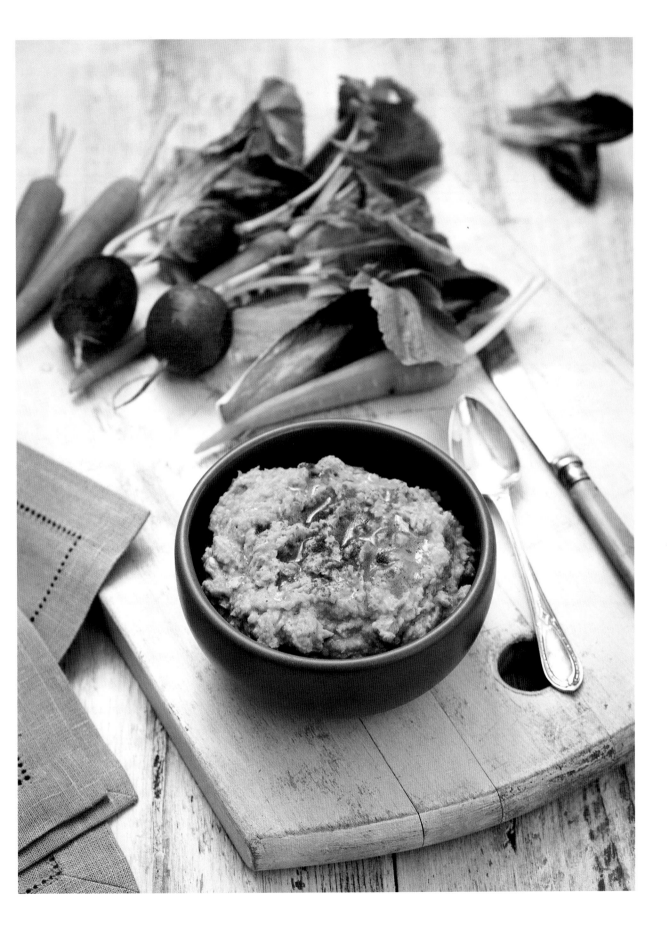

PAD THAI OMELETTE

359 calories per omelette

We love this recipe and it makes a perfect carb-free lunch. We've kept the calories down by using carrot, courgettes and bean sprouts instead of noodles. We do allow a sprinkling of peanuts, though, as they really make a difference to the flavour. If possible, use a large frying pan, about 23cm in diameter, so you can make very thin omelettes that roll up beautifully. And do check what tamarind paste you use. If it's concentrated, use just a teaspoon, but if not you'll need about a tablespoonful. Don't be tempted to add more, as it will upset the balance of flavours.

Serves 2
Prep: 20 minutes
Cooking time: about 15 minutes

1 tbsp vegetable oil
1 shallot, sliced
1 carrot, cut into matchsticks
1 small courgette, cut into
   matchsticks
5g chunk of fresh root ginger,
   peeled and finely chopped
1 red chilli, deseeded and sliced
2 garlic cloves, sliced
100g shelled raw tiger prawns,
   roughly chopped
100g bean sprouts
oil, for spraying
4 eggs
flaked sea salt
freshly ground black pepper

Sauce
1 tsp tamarind paste (1 tbsp if it's
   not concentrated)
1 tbsp fish sauce
1 tsp palm sugar (or caster sugar)
¼ tsp shrimp paste (optional)

To serve
2 spring onions, shredded
handful of coriander, chopped
1 tsp finely chopped peanuts

To make the sauce, mix all the ingredients together. Taste a little and adjust the quantities of any of the ingredients to taste.

To make the pad Thai, heat the oil in a wok until smoking, then add the shallot, carrot, courgette, ginger and chilli. Stir-fry for about 3 minutes until the vegetables are starting to cook through, then add the garlic. Stir-fry for another minute, then push everything to one side of the wok and add the prawns. Cook for another minute and then pour over the sauce. Let it bubble for a few moments and stir in the bean sprouts. Set it aside and keep warm.

Lightly spray a large non-stick frying pan with oil and place it over a medium heat until hot. Break 2 eggs into a bowl and whisk, then season with salt and pepper. Pour the eggs into the frying pan, swirling it around so the whole base is covered. Cook for a couple of minutes until the eggs are just about cooked through, then turn down the heat.

Put half of the pad Thai mixture in a line slightly to the side of the centre of the omelette. Sprinkle over half the spring onions, coriander and peanuts. Fold one side over the filling, then fold the other side over. Now roll the omelette over and out of the frying pan straight on to a plate. Repeat this with the other 2 eggs and the rest of the filling to make the second omelette and serve at once.

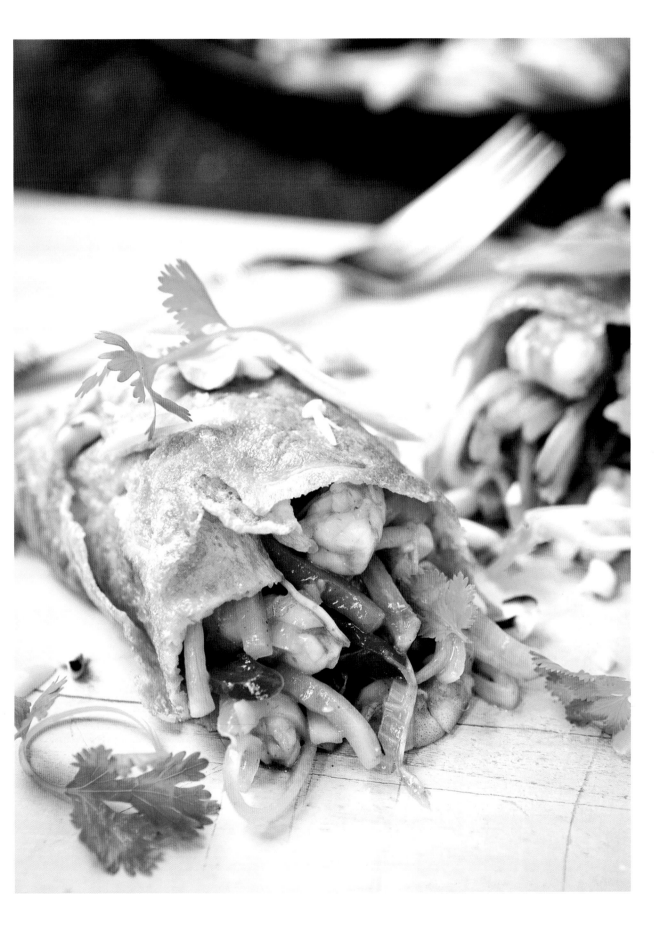

CRISPY CAULIFLOWER NUGGETS

130 calories per portion (if serving 4)

These crispy cheesy little morsels make a scrumptious starter or a snack to nibble on with a beer – and they are cheeringly low in calories. They're easy as anything to put together, but take care to drain the cauli carefully and watch that the breadcrumb mix doesn't get sticky or it will clump together and not coat properly.

Serves 4 as a starter or more
as a snack
Prep: 10 minutes
Cooking time: about 17 minutes

½ cauliflower, broken into small
    florets
6 tbsp low-fat natural yoghurt
75g very fine, dry breadcrumbs,
    such as Japanese panko
25g Parmesan cheese, finely grated
½ tsp paprika
1 tsp dried oregano or mixed herbs
oil, for spraying (optional)
flaked sea salt
freshly ground black pepper

Preheat the oven to 200°C/Fan 180°C/Gas 6. Line a baking tray with non-stick baking parchment.

Bring a large saucepan of water to the boil. Add some salt, then the cauliflower florets and blanch them for 2 minutes. Drain thoroughly and leave to dry in a colander until cool.

Put the yoghurt in a shallow bowl and mix the breadcrumbs, cheese, paprika and herbs in another bowl or plate.

Dip the cauliflower florets, a few at a time, into the yoghurt, then into the breadcrumb mixture. Toss them lightly until they are well coated with the breadcrumbs, then place them on the baking tray, spacing them out evenly. Give them a light spray of oil if you like, but this is not essential.

Bake the nuggets in the oven for 15 minutes until the coating is crunchy and starting to char slightly. Serve at once.

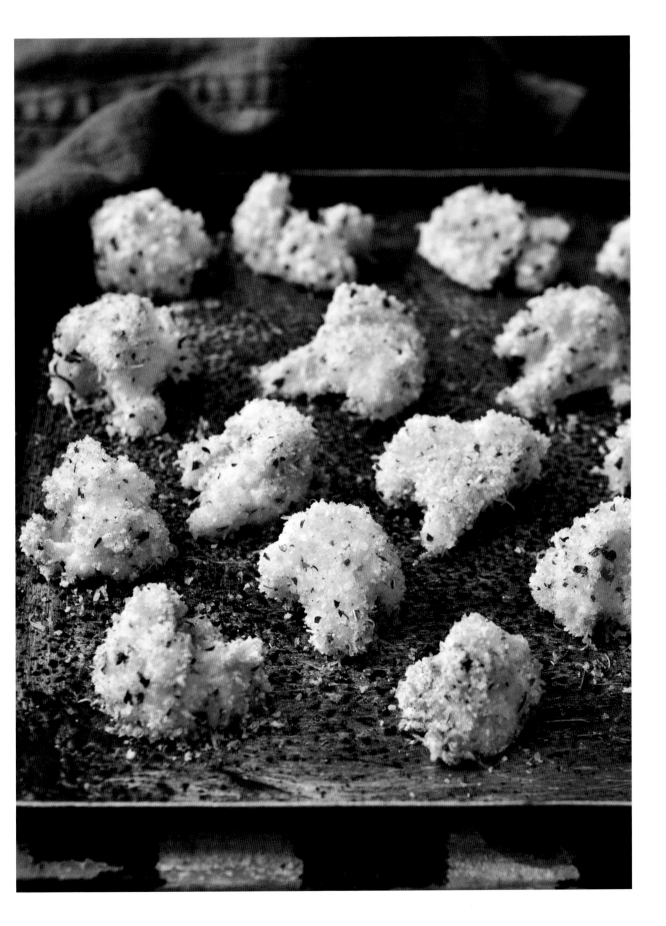

SWEET TREATS

More and more, we're realising that cutting down on sugar is just as important as keeping our fat intake under control, but like all our chums out there with a sweet tooth we don't need to despair. We've made our latest puds and bakes with as little sugar as possible, with the help of the natural sweetness in fruits such as berries, pineapple and bananas. We're particularly pleased with our fruity ice lollies, which give you a lovely sweet treat for less than 50 calories each.

SUMMER PUDDING

131 calories per portion (without crème fraiche)

There's virtually no fat in this traditional British dessert and if you use good ripe fruit you don't need much sugar either. A large white sandwich loaf works a treat for the bread casing.

Serves 6
Prep: 20 minutes, plus chilling time
Cooking time: 10 minutes

oil, for spraying
6 slices of white bread, crusts removed
300g strawberries, hulled and cut up if large
200g raspberries
200g blueberries
100g redcurrants, stalks removed, plus extra to garnish if you like
1–2 tbsp caster sugar

Lightly spray a 900ml pudding basin with oil, and line it with cling film. Take a slice of bread and cut it into a round that will fit into the bottom of the basin. Cut the rest of the slices into thirds, widthways and use most of these to line the sides. Overlap them very slightly with one another and the base to ensure there are no gaps and press the bread down as much as possible. You should have a couple of slices left over to put on top of the fruit.

Put all the fruit in a saucepan and sprinkle over a tablespoon of sugar. Add 3 tablespoons of water. Heat slowly, giving the sugar time to dissolve, then simmer very gently until the fruit is lightly cooked and has given out a lot of juice. The liquid should be a deep reddish purple. Stir as little as possible to avoid breaking up the fruit – you will find that most of the raspberries will break up anyway but that's fine, as they will provide juice for the pudding. Taste for sweetness and add more sugar, a teaspoon at a time and tasting after each addition, until you are happy with the flavour.

Ladle some of the fruit juice into the bottom of the basin and allow it to soak into the bread. Then with a slotted spoon, transfer all the fruit to the pudding basin. Pour in as much of the juice as possible, without it overflowing, then top with the remaining bread. Put a saucer on top of the pudding and weight it down with something heavy, such as a can of tomatoes. Put the pudding in the fridge and leave it for several hours, preferably overnight. Save any leftover juice for covering white patches and serving with the pudding.

When you are ready to serve, place a serving plate upside-down on top of the basin and turn the basin over to unmould the pudding. Carefully peel off the cling film. Cover any white patches with leftover fruit juice and garnish with extra berries if you have some. Serve with dollops of low-fat crème fraiche, if you like, but don't forget to add the extra calories.

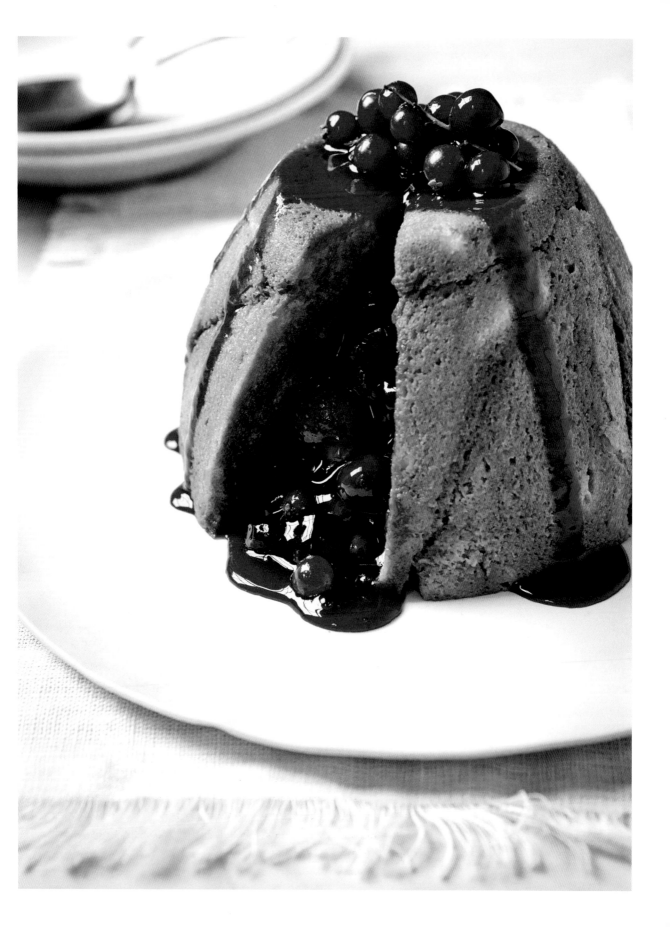

RHUBARB AND ORANGE MERINGUE TARTLETS

153 calories per tartlet

Rhubarb can be tart and sour, but if your rhubarb is nice and pink and sweet you may get away with using even less sugar. This is a clever little pud.

Serves 6
Prep: 25 minutes
Cooking time: about 40 minutes

oil, for spraying
3 sheets of filo pastry

Filling
300g rhubarb, cut into 1cm rounds
2 tbsp caster sugar
zest and juice of 1 orange
1 tsp cornflour

Meringue
2 egg whites
100g sugar
1 tsp cornflour

Preheat the oven to 190°C/Fan 170°C/Gas 5. Lightly spray 6 holes in a muffin tray with oil.

To make the filo pastry cases, cut each sheet of filo into 8 squares. Layer 4 together, by overlapping them across one another so you end up with a multi-pointed star shape. Lightly spray the centre of each case with oil and bake them in the oven for 10 minutes, until they take on some colour.

To make the filling, put the rhubarb in a large saucepan and sprinkle over the sugar and orange zest. Add 50ml of water and cover. Cook very slowly over a gentle heat until the rhubarb is soft, then remove the rhubarb from the saucepan with a slotted spoon, leaving the juice in the pan.

Add the orange juice to the rhubarb juice in the pan. Mix the cornflour with a splash of water until it is smooth and add this to the saucepan. Heat slowly, while stirring, until the liquid thickens. Tip the rhubarb back into the saucepan and mix it with the sauce, being careful not to break up the rhubarb too much. Divide the filling between the 6 tartlet cases.

To make the meringue, whisk the egg whites until they have formed stiff peaks. Mix the sugar with the cornflour and gradually add this to the egg whites until you have a thick, glossy meringue. Pile the meringue on top of the rhubarb, forming peaks. The easiest way to do this is to spoon it on, but you can pipe it if you prefer.

Bake the tartlets in the oven for 15–20 minutes, until the meringue is golden brown, but still quite soft.

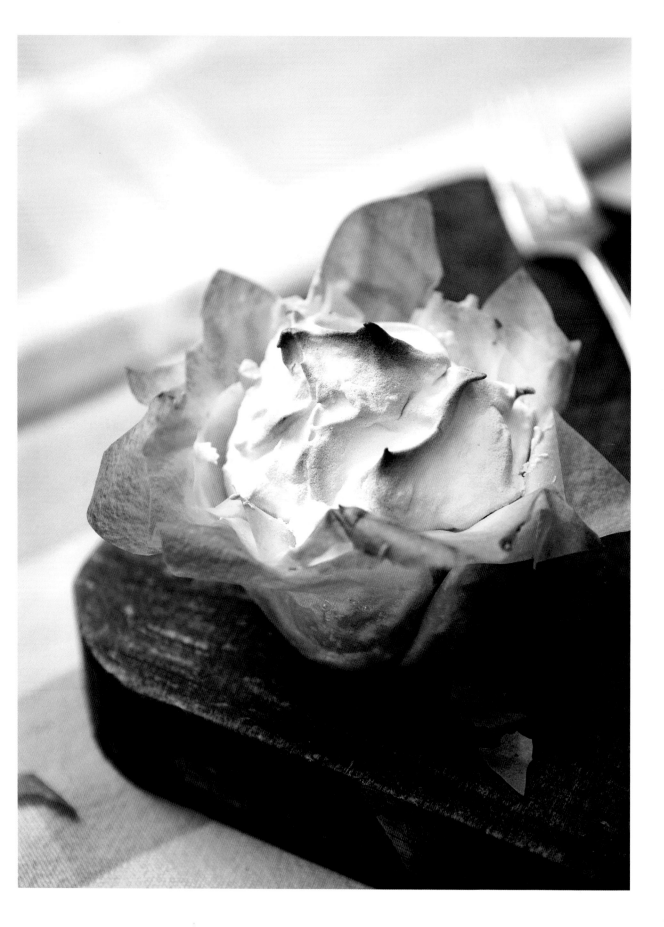

GINGER BISCUITS

58 calories per biscuit

We do like something to dunk and these are like little gingernuts, but they're quite chewy inside. The ground ginger makes them very gingery – for a milder biscuit, add just 1 teaspoonful.

Makes about 25
Prep: 10 minutes
Cooking time: 12–15 minutes

50g golden syrup
50g butter
100g light soft brown sugar
1 egg yolk
150g plain flour
½ tsp bicarbonate of soda
2 tsp ground ginger

Preheat the oven to 190°C/Fan 170°C/Gas 5. Line 2 baking trays with baking parchment.

Melt the golden syrup and butter together in a saucepan over a gentle heat. Remove from the heat and beat in the brown sugar and egg yolk.

Sift the plain flour, bicarb and ground ginger into a bowl. Add the wet ingredients and mix thoroughly. You might think the dough is too dry at first, as it will be very crumbly, but using your hands, keep working it together until it is smooth.

Roll teaspoons of the mixture (about 15g) into balls, then place them – spaced well apart, as they will spread – on the baking trays. Bake in the oven for 12–15 minutes until the biscuits are a rich golden brown and are cracked on the surface.

Remove the biscuits from the oven. They will be very soft, but don't worry, they will firm up very quickly. As soon as they are firm enough, transfer them to a cooling rack with a palette knife.

FREEZE!

The dough will freeze without any problem, and the biscuits can be frozen too. Just reheat them in the oven for a couple of minutes and then allow them to cool and crisp up again afterwards.

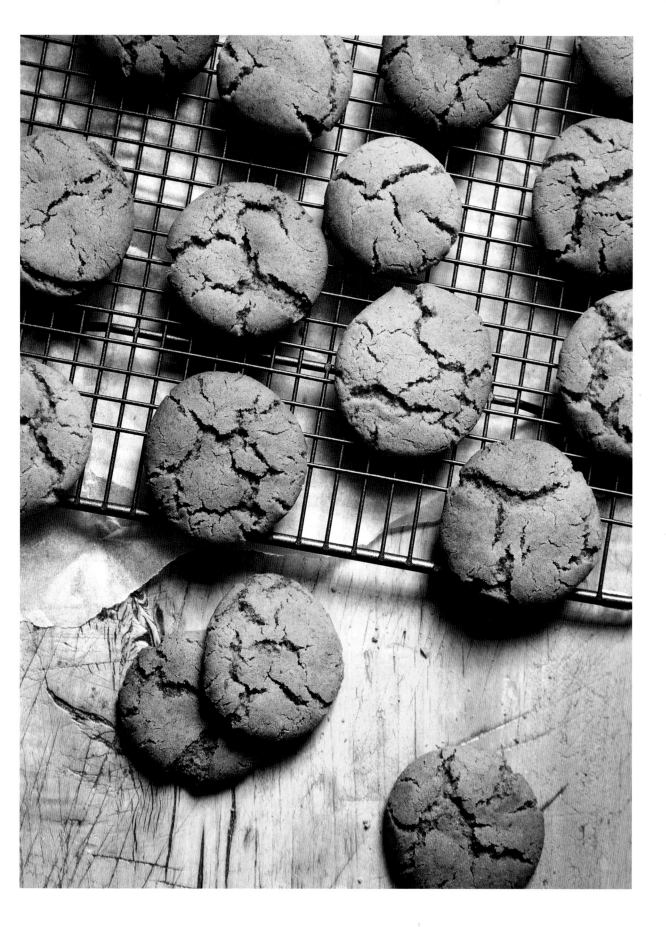

BANANA AND PINEAPPLE CAKE

205 calories per slice, if cut into 10; 171 calories per slice, if cut into 12

The banana and pineapple in this tantalisingly tropical cake keeps it lovely and moist and adds sweetness so you can keep the sugar content down. Just the thing with a cuppa to see you through to supper time.

Makes 1 cake with 10–12 slices
Prep: 20 minutes
Cooking time: 50–60 minutes

oil, for spraying
175g self-raising flour
2 tsp baking powder
½ tsp bicarbonate of soda
1 tsp grated nutmeg
75g soft light brown sugar
2 eggs
3 bananas (about 250g in weight), mashed
100g butter, melted
1 tsp vanilla extract
100g pineapple, finely diced

Preheat the oven to 180°C/Fan 160°C/Gas 4. Lightly spray the base and sides of a 2lb loaf tin with oil and line it with baking parchment.

Sift the flour, baking powder and bicarb into a large bowl and mix in the nutmeg and sugar. In a smaller bowl, beat the eggs, then add the mashed bananas, melted butter and vanilla extract. Add the egg mixture and the diced pineapple to the dry ingredients, then gently fold everything together until you have a pineapple-flecked batter.

Pour the batter into the prepared loaf tin and bake for 50–60 minutes, until a skewer comes out clean. Allow the cake to cool in the tin for 10 minutes, then transfer it to a cooling rack.

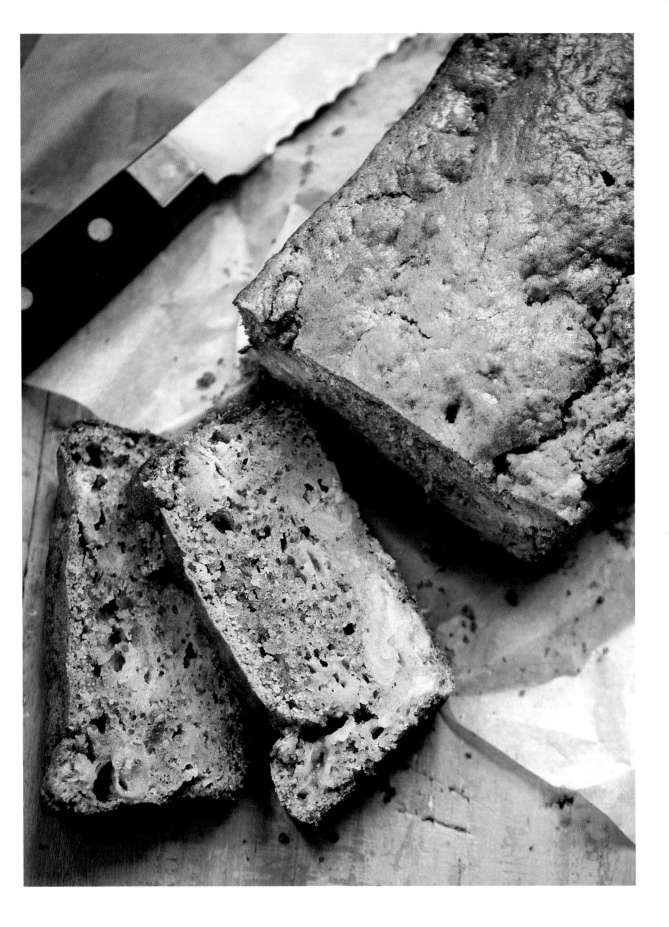

PLUM AND MAPLE SYRUP STEAMED PUDDINGS

234 calories per pudding

This makes 8 individual puddings – any leftovers can be frozen, either uncooked in the basin or cooked. Be careful not to overcook or the puddings could be dry. Lovely served with a little single cream or low-cal custard.

Makes 8 individual puddings
Prep: 20 minutes
Cooking time: 35 minutes

oil, for spraying
4 plums, stoned and diced
1 tbsp maple syrup
zest and juice of 1 orange
¼ tsp cinnamon

Sponge
175g self-raising flour
2 tsp baking powder
½ tsp cinnamon
pinch of salt
2 eggs
100g butter, melted and
   slightly cooled
100g maple syrup

Lightly spray 8 small pudding basins with oil. Preheat the oven to 190°C/Fan 170°C/Gas 5.

Put the plums in a small saucepan with the syrup, orange zest and juice and the cinnamon. Simmer over a medium heat until the plums have softened, but not broken down. Divide the plums and syrup between the pudding basins.

Sift the self-raising flour, baking powder and cinnamon into a large bowl, add a pinch of salt and stir well. In a separate bowl, beat the eggs, then add the butter and maple syrup. Pour the wet ingredients into the dry ingredients and mix thoroughly, then divide between the pudding basins.

Put the puddings in a roasting tin and pour in just-boiled water to come halfway up the sides of the basins. Bake in the preheated oven for 20–25 minutes.

Carefully remove the puddings from the hot water. Run a knife round the inside of each basin to release the pudding, then turn out on to serving plates. Great with single cream or low-cal custard.

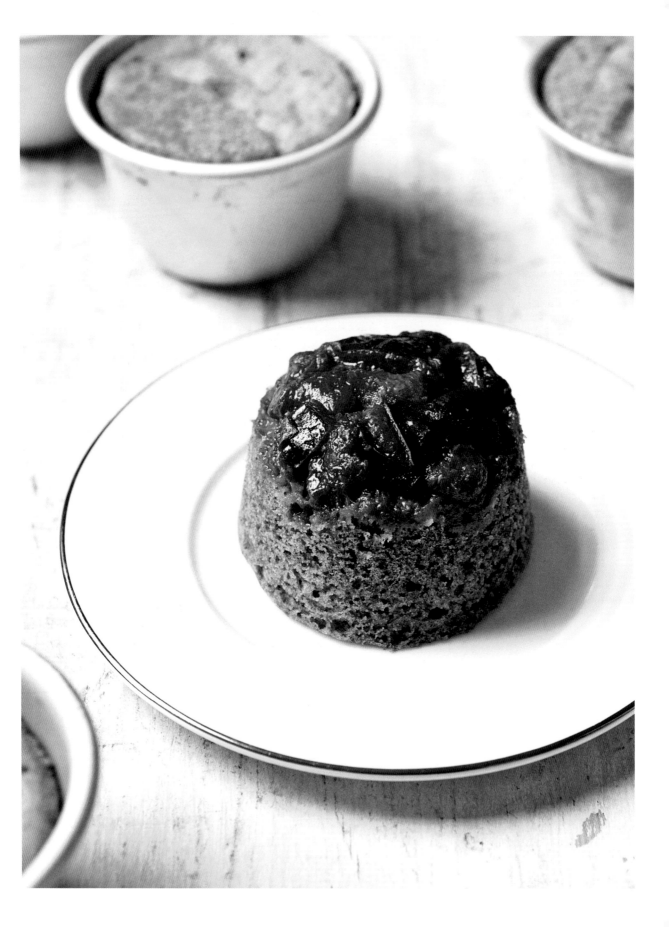

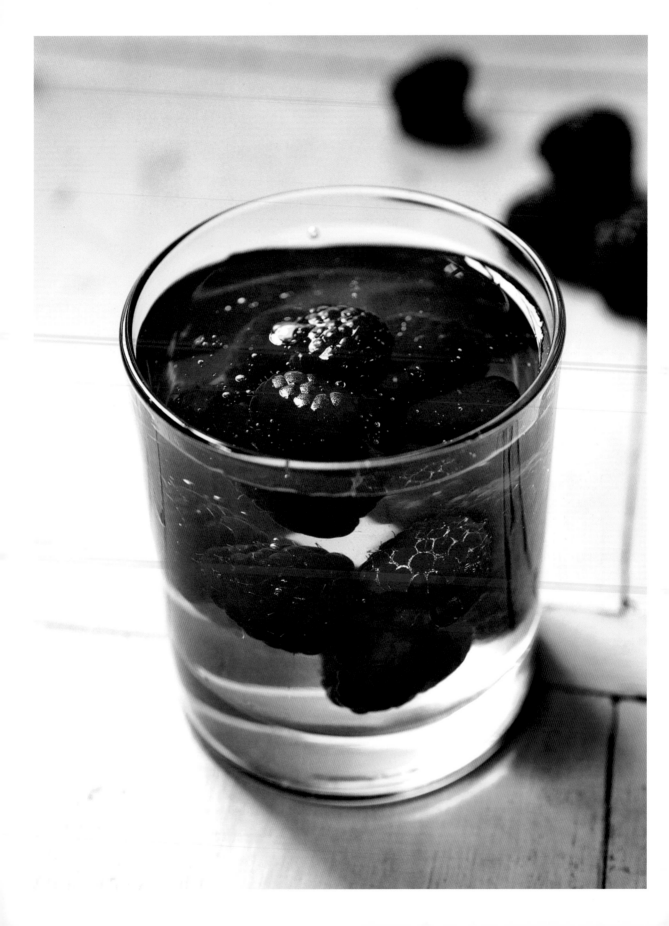

WINE, ELDERFLOWER AND RASPBERRY JELLIES

153 calories per portion

*Jellies for grown-ups, these are easy to prepare and they look and taste fab.
We don't think it matters much if the fruit isn't evenly distributed, but we've
given a few tips below if you want to try.*

Pour the wine and cordial into a saucepan, add the sugar and heat until the sugar has dissolved. Put the sheets of gelatine in a bowl of cold water and leave them to soak until they've softened. Drain and wring out the gelatine, then add it to the wine mixture. Stir over a low heat until the gelatine has dissolved, but be careful not to let the mixture boil.

Strain the mixture into a jug. Divide the fruit between 4 glasses and pour over the wine mixture. Chill the jellies in the fridge until set – this should take 3–4 hours – or leave them overnight.

If you want an even distribution of the fruit you can stir the jelly every few minutes until it is almost set. Or, you can assemble the jellies in thirds: divide a third of the fruit between the glasses, top with the jelly mixture and allow to set in the fridge, then repeat the process twice more until you've used all the mixture.

Serves 4
Prep: 10 minutes, plus setting time

400ml white or sparkling wine
100ml elderflower cordial
1 tbsp caster sugar
5 sheets of leaf gelatine
200g raspberries

BAKED PEACHES

269 calories per portion without amaretto; 241 per portion with amaretto

Some peaches are sweet and delicious just as they are, but others need a little help and this recipe does the trick. The tiny bit of honey adds just enough sweetness. We don't think there's any need to skin the peaches and there's a danger of them collapsing if skinned.

Serves 4
Prep: 10 minutes
Cooking time: 25 minutes

4 peaches, cut in half and
   stones removed
4 tsp honey
2 tbsp chopped almonds
8 amaretti biscuits
25g butter, melted
8 tsp amaretto liqueur (optional)

Preheat the oven to 200°C/Fan 180°C/Gas 6. Put the peaches, cut side up, in an ovenproof dish or baking tray.

Drizzle a teaspoon of honey over each of the peach halves, then put them in the oven and bake for 10 minutes.

Put the almonds in a dry frying pan and cook them over a medium heat until very lightly toasted. Crush the amaretti biscuits until they resemble coarse breadcrumbs and mix them with the almonds. Pour over the butter and mix together.

Remove the peaches from the oven. Divide the nut and biscuit mixture between the peach halves and drizzle over the liqueur, if using. Bake for another 15 minutes until the peaches and topping are lightly brown. Spoon over any cooking juices and serve with low-fat crème fraiche if you like – but don't forget to add the extra calories to your total.

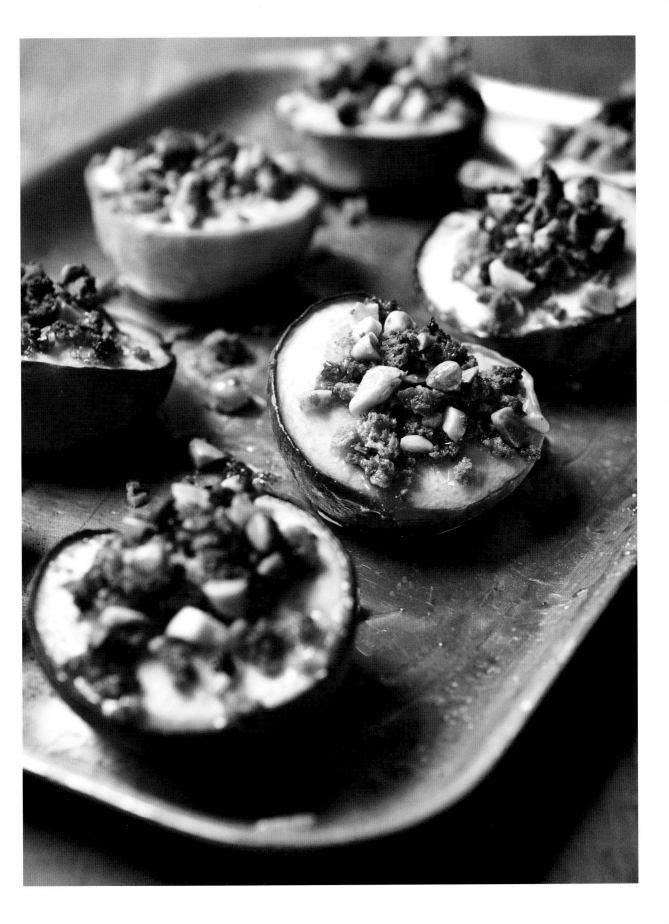

ICE LOLLIES

We made these in ice lolly trays with six holes, each holding about 50ml, but you can use any moulds you like – or even ice cube trays.

150ml reduced-fat coconut milk
150g fresh or canned pineapple
1 tbsp rum or Malibu
1 tbsp honey or sugar (optional)

PINA COLADA ICE LOLLIES

44 calories per 50ml lolly

Pineapples vary enormously in sweetness so you may or may not need to add honey to this.

Put the coconut milk, pineapple (drained, if using canned), and the rum or Malibu in a blender and blitz until smooth. Taste for sweetness and add some sugar or honey if you think it needs it, then blitz again. Spoon off any foam and pour the liquid into moulds or ice cube trays and freeze until set.

100ml fat-free natural yoghurt
1 banana (about 100g peeled weight)
juice of ½ lime
100g blueberries
a few drops of vanilla extract
1 tbsp honey

BLUEBERRY, BANANA AND YOGHURT ICE LOLLIES

45 calories per 50ml lolly

Put the yoghurt, banana, lime juice and half the blueberries in a blender with the vanilla and honey. Blend until fairly smooth – there'll probably still be some flecks of blueberry but that's fine. Add the remaining blueberries and pulse a couple of times to break them up roughly. Pour into moulds or ice cube trays and freeze until set.

200g strawberries
juice of 1–2 oranges (about 100ml)
juice of ½ lime
2 tbsp sugar

STRAWBERRY AND ORANGE ICE LOLLIES

35 calories per 50ml lolly

Put everything in a blender and blitz until smooth. If you want to get rid of the strawberry seeds, sieve the mixture before pouring it into your moulds or ice cube trays, then freeze until set.

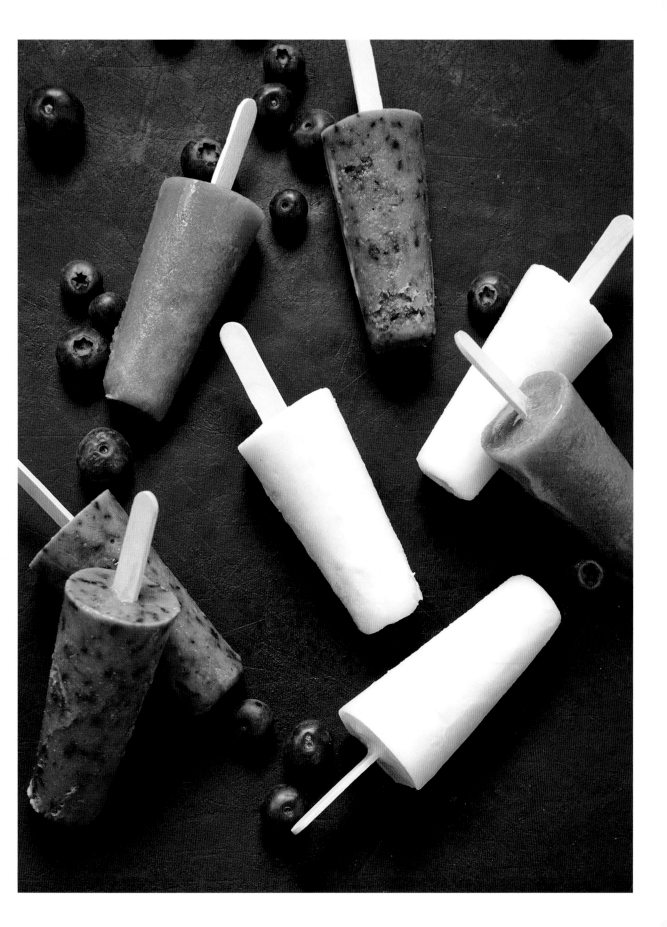

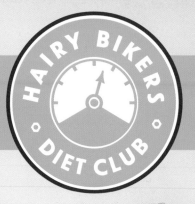
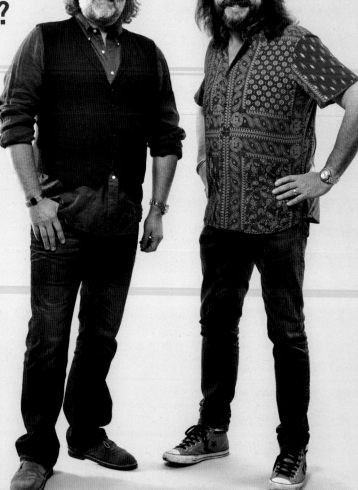
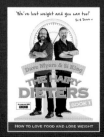
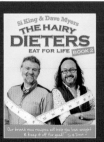

INDEX

A BIG ROUND OF APPLAUSE!

We love writing our books but we couldn't do it without all the
wonderful help and support from Team Hairy.

First of all we'd like to thank Catherine Phipps for her fantastic help and advice on the recipes, and Professor
Ashley Adamson and Dr Suzana Almoosawi of the Institute of Health & Society and Human Nutrition
Research Centre, Newcastle University, for their guidance on nutrition and for answering all our crazy questions.

Mega thanks to Andrew Hayes-Watkins who took all the photographs and always makes everything
look so tempting and beautiful. He's a special talent. And we're eternally grateful to Lisa Harrison,
Anna Burges-Lumsden and their assistants for preparing all the food so superbly for the pictures,
and to Loulou Clark for finding all the great dishes and pans.

Lovely Loulou has also done an amazing job on the design so big thanks to her, to Andy Bowden for his
technical assistance and to creative director Lucie Stericker. Amanda Harris, our fabulous publisher, continues
to give us huge support and encouragement and thank you too to Jinny Johnson, our editor, for helping us
string the words together. Last but not least, we'd like to thank our Diet Club members for all their ideas
and feedback – we've all learned that dieting need never be boring. We love you all.

As always we would like to express our appreciation to all at James Grant Mangement who are always
there for us. Big hugs to Nicola Ibison, Natalie Zietcer, Tessa Findlay, Rowan Lawton and
Eugenie Furniss – you're the best and we can't thank you enough. We'd also like to thank the
Optomen team who worked so hard on the original Hairy Dieters television series.